Quantum

Healing

Power of Self-healing and Laws of Quantum

(Unlocking the Hidden Potential of Energy Medicine Self-healing through the Laws of Quantum Physics)

Patrick Jones

Published By **Simon Dough**

Patrick Jones

Quantum Healing: Power of Self-healing and Laws of Quantum (Unlocking the Hidden Potential of Energy Medicine Self-healing through the Laws of Quantum Physics)

ISBN   978-1-9995502-5-7

No part of this guidebook shall be reproduced in any form without permission in writing from the publisher except in the case of brief quotations embodied in critical articles or reviews.

Legal & Disclaimer

The information contained in this book is not designed to replace or take the place of any form of medicine or professional medical advice. The information in this book has been provided for educational & entertainment purposes only.

The information contained in this book has been compiled from sources deemed reliable, and it is accurate to the best of the Author's knowledge; however, the Author cannot guarantee its accuracy and validity and cannot be held liable for any errors or omissions. Changes are periodically made to this book. You must consult your doctor or get professional medical advice before using any of the suggested remedies, techniques, or information in this book.

Upon using the information contained in this book, you agree to hold harmless the Author from and against any damages, costs, and expenses, including any legal fees potentially resulting from the application of any of the information provided by this guide. This disclaimer applies to any damages or injury caused by the use and application, whether directly or indirectly, of any advice or information presented, whether for breach of contract, tort, negligence, personal injury, criminal intent, or under any other cause of action.

You agree to accept all risks of using the information presented inside this book. You need to consult a professional medical practitioner in order to ensure you are both able and healthy enough to participate in this program.

Table Of Contents

Chapter 1: what is a Shaman?

There are many individuals' definitions of what an Shaman is, however I'd prefer to share with the reader what Shaman to me. Shaman signifies to me. Specifically, what is a Slipstream Shaman can be. The Slipstream Shaman actively interacts with the spirit and energy of others to aid people in their healing and develop. It happens on a other level than what that which we encounter in our daily human existence.

It is also important to consider how important it is to consider the Slipstream. If you change something within the Quantum world, you don't perform a transformation that only has only a brief result. What I'm referring to as the Quantum World also known as the Quantum Room is a place it is possible to visit in which energy is converted to benefit you. When you change your mind, it will travel through time ahead and back. The Slipstream that you build during healing opens up a place that allows for other transformations to take place quickly.

The topic will be healing for seven generations. It is a process which heals those who came before you seven generations back as well as your future family members seven generations down the line. Shaman all over all over the globe view healing in more ways than an individual. It is believed that the Haudenosaunee (Iroquois) are able to heal seven generations ago, and they help the Maori in New Zealand heal seven generations both in the past, in addition to seven generations into the future. Within the Quantum Room time behaves differently it is not a linear process we are used to.

Reconciliation, change of behavior love, forgiveness, and many other aspects will enter the Slipstream to bring about massive changes. The Slipstream flows with great speed, allowing us to change our lives effortlessly!

My Journey

I've always had an interest in things that don't necessarily fit with what is expected of me. My involvement in the Quantum Room isn't any different. I believe that there's more to the universe than what I am able to touch and be able to comprehend. The movies I watched about science fiction and reading books about science fiction made me want to know more about the world and discover the other information available beyond the contents of medical books and self-help guides.

I was looking into ways of expanding my awareness. I was interested in having an experience that was out of body. I wanted to see astral projection and remote view. I longed to enjoy vivid dreams each the night! The amazing and magical activities that other people were performing and I wanted to try also. I've participated with training in each of these fields; however they haven't worked for me on a regular basis.

In 2007, I was contacted by the Slipstream Shaman to take part in a energetic training. My experiences with this individual triggered my development to what I am now calling becoming an Slipstream Shaman. When I was working on energy work and meditation, I had another idea in my head. What's my goal? Uncertainty about my mission has affected me. How do I become an effective leader if I do not have a clear idea of my goals? Do I harm me, my family and everyone else in the absence of knowing what my goal is but not doing anything about the idea? What is my mission?

It was a blessing that while I did the work on energy the thoughts of my brain would decrease as well as my attention increase. While studying my interaction with the energy field, I noticed that words were manifesting through my thoughts. To Help. My purpose was clear! There was nothing grand, nothing deep or complicated. The goal was to help.

The thing I wasn't aware of that time ago I didn't, and perhaps don't really grasp the significance of "To Help" is a huge motive. In the way I've come realize, it is to help myself, aid other people, assist animals, aid the planet or even assist the Universe. These two phrases that appear easy are actually huge opportunities to make life more effective.

As I look back, I recognize that I've been trying to understand my mission and working towards implementing my mission "To Help" for many years. I was studying Neural Linguistic Programming (NLP), Emotional Freedom Technique (EFT) frequently called tapping as well as Hypnosis. The various modalities I had studied had led me to Help.

The majority of the methods I utilize within The Quantum Room have their genesis through techniques utilized to perform NLP, EFT, and the practice of hypnosis.

The process of learning how to harness the power of energy in The Quantum Room has been the means for me to become immersed in my goal as well as "To Help."

Through the many years of the process of learning to operate within the Quantum Room I've helped many animals and people. The majority of these experiences are discussed on the pages to follow. The names will not be shared as well as keep all information confidential.

When you are reading Slipstream Shaman You may think that the methods within this book are too quick. Particularly if you've studied old-fashioned methods for finding your spirit animal or spirit guides. A lot of these methods are lengthy and drawn-out processes including sleep deprivation eating fasts, and various other techniques. If you'd like to follow a traditional method rather that is not discussed in this book take the time to do. It's crucial for you to choose the best option for you. Engage your instructor to get maximum benefit from any course.

The processes that were that were developed by Shaman hundreds of thousands of years ago occurred in a slow time. Although there was the pressure on individuals and communities, they were not in a rush; they did not have the burden due to many of the "conveniences" that have sped our lives. No phones, no vehicles, no internet, no spreadsheets. The world was much simpler in the past and both the Shaman and the patient could have longer time to focus on to complete the task. It's crucial to discover your ideal place. You can take as much time as you want, then be at your pace.

- Some basic information before we begin

Get a journal. Make use of whatever is best for your needs. I prefer a spiral notebook. If you would prefer a leather-bound journal, go for it. If you own a hardbound journal, you can use it. If electronic journals are the best option for you, make use of it. It is always awe-inspiring to review my work at how most of what I'm unable to remember. When you are working on fears, traumas as well as other personal problems and issues, you'll be surprised at the amount of information you can't think about. Things that dominated the majority of your thinking have become a blurred memory. It is important to keep a record of your successes, and keep the joy that comes from helping someone to improve the quality of their life. Make sure to keep a record and your future self will be grateful!

The first step is with learning to tap into our energy, and then to put it on our bodies to safeguard ourselves. Your energy will protect yourself, your family, friends relatives, as well as the people whom you help. If you are a believer, it can help many others seek the help of a god for security. It will be interesting to discover the power of your belief system and how you can use your faith to protect yourself as well as guidance.

As you improve your skills, you'll encounter numerous "coincidences". It took me a long time before I believed that I could help people. I would assist someone with an problems and I would consider:

Perhaps she got over her nightmares, and it occurred at the same time I worked with her.

Perhaps her medication for heart health helped her instead of just treating a sign

It is possible that his heart is stronger than doctors are able to measure He may continue to be alive.

Perhaps the liver of the dog just suddenly started working properly in a new way

Perhaps his prostate wasn't affected in the end and his testing was flawed on during the first test

I couldn't even admit to myself that I had helped. I still struggle taking credit. I'm a conduit to facilitate the process of recovery. Make a commitment to aid, and consider yourself an integral component of the solution. More than you can ever imagine.

In the course of time, these coincidences began to pile in. I started to think that I had helped. Never have I been as content as in helping somebody recover. It's a great feeling to be rewarded internally.

Chapter 2: Becoming a Shaman

I was unaware I was transforming into an Shaman when I began to learn various ways to assist me and others. In truth, at the time I didn't know what the term Shaman was. I'd seen them in the television as well as in films with a poncho, or animal skins with rattles and potions. In a state of trance, they were casting spells. Now I know this is not the only thing is a Shaman is doing or being (thanks Hollywood). Although there are some Shamans are dressed in this manner and perform the same behaviors and practices that are seen on TV, this isn't what I am doing. What you wear and what you wear don't make the person an actual Shaman. Your soul, your intention as well as your capacity to communicate with your spirit and energy on a the higher levels of your consciousness makes you Shaman. Shaman.

Being Shaman to me, being a Shaman involves using meditation to take my mind into an altered state in which I can interact with the energy of my surroundings and assist animal and human beings, the communities, and ultimately the entire planet. The altered state is the place I've named the Quantum Room. This will all be explored in more depth further in the book. The book will also include hyperlinks that will direct you to video clips of me working these processes, and demonstrating the way I do it.

Although I could aid many people using NLP, EFT and Hypnosis but I did not officially begin the process of becoming Shaman Shaman until I was able to discover my own energy. Once I discovered my power, everything associated with the development of my own began to speed up. The creativity I had for my goal To Help grew exponentially. my enthusiasm for the topic increased, and I started to explore and obtain results that truly amazed me. It continues to amaze me.

There's the Buddhist phrase that reads "when the student is ready the instructor will appear". That was the case for me. Although at the time, I didn't know for sure the fact that To help was the goal of my life however, I was aware I had a desire to know how to aid others. But I was not sure of exactly how.

When I was thinking about the best way to proceed my friend phoned me and asked me to take part in a training in paranormal investigations that the team took part in along together with the help of a Shaman. The purpose of the course was to instruct us on the best ways to safeguard our own and those around us from demons and evil spirits.

The course was held in a an amazing setting within The Utah desert. The Shaman would be teaching you how to harness your own energy. It is my belief that we still refer to the word energy ball, even though the majority of individuals don't see their energy manifested as an actual ball. Sometime, your energy may appear as if it's an actual ball. Certain people's energy appears like the shape of a gelatinous ball, others appears like lightning, while others seem like a tiny sun. Like every snowflake or fingerprint is distinctive, every person is unique in their energy. Also, while I may call the ball energy ball, please be aware that your energy may not appear like an actual ball.

I'll be honest. This method of training was not working for my experience. The Shaman was not aware the different energy. She tried to influence her beliefs of the people she was instructing. She believed that everyone's energy should appear like hers. She was so determined on how she wanted it to look and felt that I was did not even bother with that aspect of her education.

It was a blessing that I was able to retain enough of the experience that I was able to continue working at it by myself and regain my energies. I believe having this ability was the foundation of my growth as Shaman. Shaman. As I searched for my own strength, I was struck by an expression from Lao Tzu that sounds like a sequel to the Buddhist phrase, "when the student is prepared, the teacher shows up. If the student truly at the point of readiness, the teacher disappears". This was the case for myself. With no teacher who was talking about her view of what was going on I was able to get my energy back and accomplish amazing things using it.

Connecting with our own energy can be a good place to begin our journey. Energy is the foundation and the foundation of our growth. It is the energy you use to move through time. Your energy will be used to safeguard your spiritual security. Your energy will be used to attain the abundance. Your energy will be used to strengthen your connections to people, both individuals as well as a group. The energy you generate will serve to draw positive energy into your life.

There are many reasons to possess something that can assist you in the direction of your goals. Many have utilized crystals, rocks as well as rattles, sticks, along with other things to serve as the talisman that helps focus and direct your energy. I've created many rattles myself as well as for others. There are many people that I have met who utilize crystals and rocks.

As you contemplate the power of an occult talisman, what do you think of? Does anything pop out? Do you envision the idea of a stone, a stick perhaps, or a rattle, or other thing you feel could assist you? If yes, then start planning what you'd like to do with it. Perhaps, you do not require the item. All of us are on our individual journey. Explore, think, and consider what might be most effective for you. I am in love with rattles, and make often for my relatives and friends. If you have something could be used as an occult talisman, I would like to encourage you to play around and build your skills with the rattle.

This is the time to have fun! It is time to discover how to harness your own energy. There is a belief that small chakras are located inside your palms hands. These chakras are the place where my energy is manifested and I have seen my students achieve similar results. Make sure to do your breathing prior to starting. Relax in a position that feels comfortable, and permits the body to take in enough oxygen without straining. Relax your eyes and concentrate on your breathing for five minutes. Breathe in for a number of four, hold the breath to a number of 4. Breathe out in a 4 count and keep your lungs empty for the duration of four. In 5 minutes, you'll be ready to tap into the energy you have stored up.

Keep in mind that this is your experience your experience is valuable. Allow the energy to manifest and manifest, do not try to force it, or establish an exact timeframe, just feel. There's no right or wrong method for that energy's manifestation. It may be of any color and could be mixed shades. It may be any shape and have any type of type of texture. Its temperature can be unique to all of us. My energy is extremely cold to the touch however; most of my students report that they feel warm, and even scorching. I'm writing this to the people who are like you. Enjoy!

Access your energy.

Sit down, get comfortable, close your eyes, open your heart

Place your hands shoulders apart, with your the palms facing one another. Be comfortable; keep your hands in a position that will not make you tired.

A few people choose to place their pelvis and chest over each other, instead of to either side. Use your hands in the way that feels the best your choice, just use it in a way it feels comfortable for you.

Concentrate on the area between your palms, and then gradually move your hands towards each other.

How do you feel when you pull them closer to one another? Hot, warm, cool, cold? Every person's energy is different.

Are you able to see a color within your fingers? It doesn't matter what color you see that is, it's the color you are as well as the possibility of multiple colors to be a sign of your energetic flow

How does energy appear like? Do you think it looks like the sun shining energy? Do you see an unsettling mass? Do you think it looks like it's solid? There's no correct or wrong way to appear - it's the energy you put into it.

Your hands should move between your hands at a slow pace. The energy will build, and you'll get focused. What is it like to feel? Are you able to smell or taste it? Spend a couple of minutes engaging your energy and having fun with it.

Then, practice the movement. Give it to a loved one or pet. It is pure love and they'll love it!

Find out how much you create it. Can you cover yourself? Are you able to allow it completely cover the area you're within? Are you able to make it completely be a part of your city? Can you cover your state? Are you able to cover the Earth? Are you able to touch the whole universe?

Take some time to relax and enjoy the energy. It's been there all the time. the loop, but now you know about it.

As with a muscular muscle, your capacity to utilize your energy effectively and think creatively using the energy you have will require practice. Working with and utilizing your power is an excellent opportunity to recharge and relax. The combination of it can be a great way to mindfulness and enjoy an enjoyable activities at any point of the day. Don't operate or drive unsafe equipment when you are meditating. It will be clear that this is among your most relaxing and enjoyable practice you've ever experienced. Take your time!

Chapter 3: Some of my Daily Energy Work

My morning routine is to concentrate on my health and to protect my body from it. It is my intention to create security, positivity, and abundant wealth. This allows me to be motivated for my day! When you practice this, notice the increased oxygen flowing through you, filling the cells of all your cells.

After I've completed my physical body's coverage, the next thing I focus to send my energies to loved ones and further. My energy is sent to my home and all of my family members. I then extend that energy into the area they reside in as well as sometimes expanding the coverage of my nation and the whole world. Maybe you can increase your energy up to the dimensions of a galaxy? Find out how far you could expand your reach.

If you use your energies, think creatively Use your imagination and you'll be amazed by what you can accomplish! This illustrates the way I utilize my energy to protect myself. In my youth, I was reading a science-fiction tale that was set in a different planet. If it was the an appropriate time for the protagonist to go to bed the character would put cubes in the area where he'd rest. They would create the shape of a forcefield surrounding him, providing security while he slept and insecure. If I'm getting ready for go to bed and I feel that something isn't good, I protect myself by covering my body with energies to shield myself, and then I instantly relax and feel comfortable.

On a paranormal research I met a person who advised us to protect ourselves from negativity. I gathered my energy in my fingers and wrapped my body in the energy. I said to it that I wanted it to help my body. Since then I practice this everyday. In the mornings and at times in the evening, at times both.

The energy I channel into my body is a wonderful feeling and I also believe that this, in addition to protecting me is a source for energy and cleansing to my entire body. I'll wrap myself with my radiant energy and let it be reflected through my body to cleanse impureness, killing sickness as well as energizing my cells. I feel more confident, healthier and more assured whenever I allow my body to feel this energizing power.

At times, I'll be able to stand up and let the power of the sun shine through my body. I wish it could go through every cell in order to rid it of any impurities. Every cell needs to get nourishment from Quantum energy and to be in good health! It's beautiful. I feel every cell getting stronger and cleansing. When the energy flow is flowing throughout me, I'm giving my body the permission to let go of toxins and harmful substances that are stored.

Many things can be accomplished using this energy. One of the questions I asked myself while meditation I asked "what is this energy?". My response is "it is your energy; it is aligned with your personal vibration and it is how you manifest love".

Love is a energetic energy that is high in vibration. Take a look at times when bad things happened that energy of high vibration could assist. For instance, driving. Ich will be honest and admit that I'm a very irritable driver. At times I am annoyed when drivers change lanes to make me angry. They speed up or decrease speed just to bother me. There are a myriad of ways that drivers go about their business to make me angry. I began to manifest my energy ball and putting it along the road I was planning to take. I requested the energy ball to ensure an enjoyable and safe drive. Making that intention positive and then directing that energy to the future to assist me on my journey is helping me become a more comfortable and relaxed driver. Families and friends might advise me to practice this more frequently.

Another area to apply your energy is to help someone that is unhappy. If you see someone getting angry and you'd like to help. Perhaps a hug could help or maybe just a nice phrase, or perhaps you can send affection to this individual. Send an influx of love and affection to someone struggling. Allow the love to be a part of them. Let it flow throughout them and take in by them. It will show a difference in their attitude even without telling that you shared your love with them.

Are you able to think of instances where a child was having an issue? This could be the child of a friend's child, or a friend or even a stranger. Let your love radiate from you and observe what happens. Do they feel relaxed? Do they pay attention, and do you see them smiling? There are many wonderful outcomes that can occur when you offer your affection with a child suffering from distress.

Cats, dogs as well as horses and chickens be a lot of fun and grow by sending your enthusiasm and your love. Everyone loves to be in connections This is a wonderful opportunity to express what you want this world. Send them joy and love. convey your conviction that they're beautiful and awe-inspiring.

It is so easy to neglect to look after our own needs? This is a tip to do at the meal time. Be focused on your energy levels, make it your goal to ensure to discover the nutrients you require at this moment. Allow your energy to choose the food you eat for lunch, breakfast, or even your dinner. Create the intention that the energy will tell you what foods to consume and what portion will provide you with the maximum energy

This is just one example of the options. There are thousands, and likely million of ways to utilize your energies to improve your lifestyle or your family's life, as well as the world a better place. Allow your imagination and creative juices to fly! You aren't limited for you to explore when riding the slipstream! Share your creations and with our Slipstream community. www.slipstreamshaman.com

The above items are just ideas. I am excited to learn what the Slipstream community will use their energies! Share your success, share your creativity, share your adventure!

Create your Quantum Room

When I'm dealing with my own personal issues or helping others, I complete the work in My Quantum Room. The space I use for my Quantum Room looks like a room that is filled with my enthusiasm as grey swirling mist forms the edges of this space. The design of your Quantum Room does not need to have this look it is likely to not appear as similar to the one in my Quantum Room.

A few examples of others' Quantum Room:

A stunning pond is safe to swim in as well as enjoy the air as you breathe in the water

A meadow that is surrounded by trees

A rocky cave

A top of a mountain

A crater in the Moon I love this image

In the water, you will find a slow-moving Kelp

A dunes made of sand.

A room made of metallic material, thought to be the spaceship

Inside a microscopic bubble

The sun's core

A parlor which appears to be from the eighteenth century. English Royalty

The interior of a vehicle

Amid Space in the middle

Your space will be constructed by your choices. I'd like to suggest that you create the space you want to create with no intention of what it might become. Simply let it happen Let it flow. No room is superior to others, your room you choose to use is just right for you. It is likely to change with you as you mature and grow.

Start making Your Quantum Room:

Lay down or sit in a position that allows you to allow you to be at ease for a lengthy duration. There is a chance that you'll spend for the next half hour or so on one spot So, be sure to feel comfortable.

Make sure you are in a good position to tap into your energy, and get started on working towards bringing your enthusiasm to others.

For a couple of minutes, breathe in four count the air, then hold for four minutes after which you can breathe out for four times and then hold breath for four counts until your lungs are empty. Hold the count of four.

If you are relaxed and have access to your energetic state, you have achieved you are able to connect with the Quantum Room. Quantum Room

Do not try to force it Relax and let the Quantum Room come to you

There is a feeling that you need to go into the area. It will happen by your thought process, and not physically.

It's possible to feel as if that you are flying into your Quantum Room

It's possible that you're swimming to the depths of your Quantum Room

You can access your Quantum space in the manner which is best for you.

Have fun, and get there to you Quantum Room at your own pace

Once you have entered the Quantum Room, I would suggest that you take the time to become familiar with the room. While I'm in my Quantum Room I am usually standing. Sometime I lie or sit down. There aren't any rules. follow your own preference and what is right for you.

What are you seeing? What do you smell? Do you notice a high or low illumination? Are there breezes or waves moving? Allow all your senses to take part. Explore the space, feel the space.

A few of you are going need to dedicate one or two days perhaps, or even days and weeks learning about the Quantum Room. Others want to go straight to work in to help others as well as themselves. Your only correct answer will be the one you choose. The most effective way to progress is to go according to your own pace. If you would like to sit inside the Quantum Room for a short period of time, and not do anything other than it, then go for it. The way that feels best to you is the best choice.

Once I walked into that I had a Quantum Room I just sat down and let myself get familiar with the space. The majority of the time, what's happened for me within my Quantum Room has been instinctual. This means that my instincts was telling me the right thing to do. I knew exactly what I needed to do. I was back home.

In the beginning, when I was first granted access to the Quantum Room I used it to heal myself. It provided a sanctuary where I could unwind in reflection, and to get my thoughts out. The last few months, the Quantum Room was a just for me. Like many readers of this book, there was lots to heal, and lots to deal with. It was an amazing and safe space for me to tackle my difficulties and to become a better person. It wasn't clear to me that it would become a place in which I could aid other people.

In the beginning I was unaware that I'd never be able to recall the events that took place within the Quantum space unless I note it down. There is a reason why I'm unable to recall memories that have led me to meditation within Quantum and helping other people. I strongly suggest to keep an account of your journey during your time in Quantum to ensure that you don't go through any of the great moments.

I've never been able to remain in a solitary position. When I was a child, I was a runner. My interests and thoughts are always swiftly changed. Go, go, go! I still remember as a tiny child hearing my mother tell me, "that boy has ants in his pants!" when I was rushing through the day. One of my dear friends suffers from the same condition. She says it causes "Grrr". This seemed like the perfect description of how I felt within. I've struggled with focus throughout my life. If I'm in the Quantum area, I'm more relaxed but I wanted something else that could help me concentrate and that's when I began with rattles.

As I was contemplating while working in Quantum the idea came to me the head to make a rattle as a tool for concentration. The rhythm and its sound seemed as if it could help me. One idea that came up repeatedly came from "make a warrior rattle". A gourd was found the garage, and tied it to an old Elk antler a friend's dog discovered. After I had assembled my rattle, as well as using the rattle I noticed that my thoughts seemed more structured and coherent.

The thought of constructing an acoustic warrior rattle was always coming up to me. Was there a reason why I wanted an oar? What is the significance? Like every time, the answer occurred to me as I was contemplating inside the Quantum Room.

In Quantum I in Quantum, I "what do the war rattles trying to say what is the message it's trying to convey? Perhaps a more appropriate question is "what is my attempt to say about the necessity of the warrior rattle?". Was I required to use the rattle in order to combat? Was I required to use the rattle to become the warrior? Did the rattle help me focus my energy and thoughts toward a fight of some sort? It was a quick answer.

As I played with the rattle, as well as asking questions I noticed an activity within the mist which surrounds the Quantum Room. In the mist, came my pet Desi! It was a gorgeous beagle that was fearless. Absolutely no rat, snake or other unwelcome dog was permitted to roam her property. Desi was incredibly affectionate to everyone; however there was a small number of animals and none of rodents. Desi could not stand up to everything that came into her territory. She was an unstoppable fighter.

Desi died within a short time before I visited the woman in my Quantum Room and we were extremely excited to meet our friends. Once we had reconnected her, she relaxed and waited with me to begin my battle.

Another pet from my past walked in the mist. It was Max! Max was the very first pet I owned as opposed to a pet belonging to the family. I bought him using the money I earned from an employment in construction during the summer when I was just 16. Max was an English springer spaniel. My very first dog was one of the English springer spaniel that was my father's dog when I was just a tiny boy. I'm incredibly attached to these dogs. Max was an absolute soldier. Max had a tremendous patience for puppies, and loved being in the company of female canines. He also enjoyed male dogs, until they attempted to demonstrate any sort of dominance after which the battle was over. The dog would not quit, did not give up, and there was and there was absolutely no possibility of surrendering. Max was gone years before and it was wonderful to see him again! Like Desi did before, Max sat down and patiently waited for me to resume the quest of the warrior.

Then a beloved uncle of mine emerged from the fog. He was an active Marine who had served in two conflicts and was quite the. A small man, but you were sure that you should not challenge his authority. Everyone who played blocks liked and loved his work. Most of us joined the Marines. We wanted to emulate his. He was an amazing human being. It was amazing to be able to connect with him on the same level! We reconnected and his feet shifted off to the side and had a play with Desi as well as Max.

Similar to what had occurred in the past, the mist began to expand and came out the character from a novel the series that I enjoyed during high school. It was a huge green Martian with four arms who was a fighter and could never be overcome. I looked up at him I nodded and then walked towards the other side of me alongside my uncle and the dogs.

What would be the next? Another dog, a acquaintance, a fictional persona? There wasn't much time to sit.

The mist started to swirl and I saw my most favorite big monster! I adored watching Saturday night horror films however, I particularly enjoyed watching the monster films which were shown during Sunday afternoons. There was a gigantic turtle that could breath flames, fly as well as travel to different planets. That was one of the best warriors to have on my side! In contrast to the other turtles who arrived at my door, the large turtle just stood there and listened.

My dog and my uncle, as well as the famous Martian as well as a gigantic turtle were my tough team! I believed that we were able to do almost anything! I was ready to assist those in need.

I could hear my family and friends chatting about physical ailments or emotional problem and request permission to assist them in the work on energy that I'd learned.

Desi has the greatest nose I have ever had in dogs. She was able to sniff any object, no matter how small. Nothing was beyond her ability to smell. In the event that I worked with someone else, I'd invite them to the Quantum Room and Desi began to sniff. Desi would discover things that were attached to people, or even within the people. When she was done with the item which was making them uncomfortable the rest of the team members was able to smash it, so that it would not be able to communicate with my client.

The process has always brought an individual the relief they needed. But, the process didn't necessarily last. Through the course of months or weeks, the problem or ailment returned. I saw this as a mistake of my own and felt very disappointed that my assistance didn't last. I thought to myself thousands of times "what am I doing wrong?". One day, as I sat in meditation within the Quantum Room the answer came to me. The nature hates vacuums; Love is essential during the course of.

I thought that since the rattle of a warrior kept me focused on the violent side of the game, that the love rattle could help to keep my attention on the positive side of the procedure. It was simple, combining walnut shells and rocks to create the sound. When I began to make the rattle, it made me feel certain that what I had done would prove much stronger and continue to be used for years.

It was time to build the love team. This would be a challenge. I've always found it easy to be a dog lover, as are others. However, the amount of people that I've been able to love up until the point I formed the team was quite restricted. The process was difficult to allow people into my life and I'd developed an extremely thick and unattractive shield to avoid being wounded. It was also difficult to express love. I was in desperate need of help. I needed someone to assist me.

I wasn't sure of what I was in for when I found myself in the Quantum Room and set the goal of creating the love team. In truth, I was not sure whether anyone or anything wanted to assist me.

The same method I employed to build the warrior team was used again. Within the Quantum Room I meditated and the next thing I did was ask for the love of my life team. Then there was a flurry of movement the mist, and out was my Aunt! She was among the most genuine people I've met. She was the sole adult that I felt loved by me. She passed away a couple of years ago and I could not have been more pleased to meet her. She gave me one her amazing hugs and I was sure it was going to go well.

Following that lovely hug, she moved to her side, and then the following member of the team walked out. The dog I had was Thomas! Like all the assistance in the group I'd receive at first it was in reality or a real individual or animal that was gone. In later times, animal and human beings would appear to aid However, at first they were the only spirits. Thomas was everyone's friend! Thomas was a lover of all humans and animals. He was a stunning and lovable pet. I was thrilled to meet him. The two of us played for about a minute and I watched numerous of his actions that I was almost crying. I really miss my pal. When we had reunited and he came over to my aunt. I let him welcome the next person on the group.

Sen. was a sweet puppy mix my family members had when I was in elementary school. She was sweet, patient and always happy. A cute face! The eyes of Sen Sen were so dark, you couldn't see her eyes, only black which appeared to last forever. Sen. was away for a long time, longer than all the pets and individuals that had stepped up to assist me. It was a joy for me to know that she was eager to contribute in helping other people. She eventually moved into the back to join my aunt as well as Thomas. The time was right for another group member.

The mist continued to swirl. I saw the silhouette of a tiny girl. The girl was unable to emerge from the fog. It was clear that she was watching us intently, eager to be a part of us. But something was holding her behind. The girl was unable to leave the dark to come closer. I was puzzled as to the reason she didn't come out to join the love team. My aunt put her hand on my shoulder and assured me that the situation was okay and the girl would be joining the team when she's ready.

It took a long time as well as some fantastic suggestions from a fellow acquaintance to allow her the opportunity to show her face. I'd see her at times at the edges in the Quantum Room. She was keen to join, but wasn't quite fully prepared.

Ten years after I first saw the tiny girl who seemed like part shadow, my mom died. There was a really strained relation, and I was never valued and buried an uneasy feeling about the previous. The last time we spoke, it was a long time ago and I believed that there was no chance to save the relationship.

When her possessions were divided among my siblings as well as me, I discovered the picture she had taken when she was a young girl with the pigtails. I'd shown the picture to a person who offered me great tips. The tiny girl sporting the adorable smile and pigtails could cause any harm to you. If you are thinking of your mother, why not imagine her as the adorable little girl who was not yet discovered and was damaged?

Sometimes it's hard to see the forests in the trees. This happens to me every day, where you are the point of something, but are unable to see clearly. When I came back inside the Quantum Room the little girl who was sat at the edges eventually came out to join the loving team. I remembered giving her a large hug, and felt an intense feeling of love which I'd never felt previously. It was by chance that I had repaired an old injury. The girl was a perfect fit and was a wonderful new addition to our love team.

As I've described, these was the first team, the love and warrior teams. These teams have become significantly more extensive since the beginning of their existence. In addition, many players will join each team for a portion animals or people that we assist.

New arrivals include my beloved dog Calvin who died a few years ago. He is normally on the love team but can be on the warriors' side if needed. My college rat Gonzo He is an extremely powerful and helpful companion. Greta is a Doberman Pincher in high school. Clyde Cat. Fonzi as well as Lavern both cats. The horses my father owned are now helping the love team and also as warriors.

A fascinating development is the fact that seven generations and forward are affected by the work that is being conducted within the Quantum Room. Future and previous generations are now helping the love and warrior teams. Consider how strong that will be! Imagine being in the company of 14 generations of loved ones and wish to see you be excellent! Its true love and protection.

I'm sure all beings who come to assist are able to feel my gratitude and affection. In the beginning I wasn't sure what the creatures and individuals that were in the Quantum Room were the spirit energies of what I was experiencing or if they represented my personal identity which I had been using during this method. While I write this post, it's clear that they're not just figments of my imagination, or a representation of my internal reality. My beloved family members both animal and human.

We will explain the method I employ to work in my Quantum Room with an example of a client I've collaborated with. I'll share a few tales of others' and animal experiences I've had the pleasure of working with. You can then to explore experiment and determine the best method for you.

My Process

I begin from my Quantum Room and announce who I'll be working alongside and invite my guests to join me. This animal or individual appears in front of me. In order to make it easy for me to understand, I'll call them "client". The client is often seen coming from the fog which surrounds Quantum Room Quantum Room or will just come right in front of me. We talk, sometimes and we meet up but sometimes we don't have any conversation. Each session is unique. When the client is settled I then inquire "who will help from the warrior team? ".

Desi is usually the first person to come out of the fog. When each member of our group comes in and we have a fun game or hug each other while we get ready to assist our client.

Once the warriors are complete, Desi will start sniffing about the patient. I'm not interested in knowing what the majority of clients' ailments are. It is common for me to know about at the very least one condition due to the fact that they approached me to seek advice. However, its best if I am able to go into the clinic without any preconceived ideas of what is required or what to do. Desi has the sharpest nose of any dog that I've encountered; nothing is able to get through her. She'll search until she discovers anything that is not within or near the person.

Desi discovers a variety of things in her customers. The objects she observes the "companion. Although many of the people she meets can be disgusting to view or consider, nearly all of them began with positive intentions and later, over time, turned into a negative experience for the person. They usually begin in an attempt to be beneficial. A few of the people Desi is removing include rags, parasites animals, rocks, sticks or worms, snakes or even aliens. There were a myriad of friends she's seen in clients. Sometimes, they are located situated on the outside of the body of the patient sometimes she has to search to find these things. She's very meticulous and does not leave any evidence of the issue.

The friends being taken away from the individual are a symbol of a issue an individual has. Often, the place of the co-worker is the exact same spot in the case of an injury for instance, an insect that has burrowed its way into the knee of a client who has knee pain. This isn't all the time. In this instance, for example one could discover a bone on your shoulder which causes headache or neck pain or even a hip issue. It doesn't matter where it is you can focus your attention on the partner.

Desi is able to identify the issues and other members of the team are able to hold Desi in place until we are able to resolve the issue.

Release of the partner from its client and its present situation is the next stage. There has been only one individual who didn't begin with positive outlook for the client. Most of the time, all companions began positive and should be treated with care and respect. A good example of a friend beginning with a positive intention:

Young boys are physically victimized and has an idea to be large, nothing would hurt him. The idea of being big is carried on and he eats a lot in an attempt to look bigger. The intention that the little boy had doesn't change or change with him the manifestation developed by a 4-year-old won't fit for a thirty-year-old. We will treat this manifestation/companion with respect and help it evolve.

It is not necessary to find out what is the reason behind the relationship. We'll identify the friend and help it grow and then release it in a way that it will be content and productive. This is more logical as we examine the healings that I've performed for others.

The idea may seem absurd; however removing a animal companion can be a difficult and loving procedure. Most of the time, Desi or others will drag their companion away. Imagine the image of a Badger or a snake pulling it out from the floor. There are occasions when the snake's companion is easily released; however, there are instances when they have to be pushed away.

When companions leave from the group, members of the warrior group can hold them to the ground until it's the right time for it to heal and develop.

When all companions have been taken away, it's now time to get them ready to heal. The process isn't always enjoyable; however it can help prepare the person for metamorphosis and healing. My giant turtle and I both send an extremely strong energetic stream of energy to the person which burns off the outside layer of the person. Once they're healthy and soft we let our loved ones take care of their needs. The debridement process is swift and assists the dog in its development.

The love team surrounds the person they are with and form an energetic field. The energy field begins in a clockwise direction until it draws healing energy from beneath the person, through them, and finally out to over them to the top. Healing energy usually has similar to the color of my energy however it's not necessarily. Sometimes it's transparent or white. Color doesn't matter.

Since this energy heals each component of the person and the person is healed, they change the shape. The rock that started out as a stone might transform into a bird flying out of sight. A dirty piece of cloth could transform into a tree, which will take it to the ideal spot it to flourish. The initial leach can turn into a stunning child who is happy to go on a run.

The companion is being released from the pain of a lifetime and allowing them to live the life is what it was designed to live. We thank you for your help to the friends!

It is now time for the patient to recover. The client should be taken to the loving team. The love team will accomplish similar things for the client as they have done for their friends. The vacuum that is caused by the removal of the companion is then healed, and then full of love energy so that nothing else will be attached to the person.

The client is in the company of the loving team. A field of energy is formed and begins to spin in a clockwise direction. Energy for healing is pumped into the body of the client, and heals them all and down to the cellular level, and above.

Then comes the most beautiful and stunning experiences I've ever seen. The client makes a smooth transition from their love-team. When the client gains further away from their group 7 generations of the future and seven generations of the past are gathered within the confines of the individual. From above, it looks like looking through the Mayan Calendar.

Seven generations aren't just "blood" family. They are also spirit families, as well as energy family. It is possible that they are part of the soul of the client. There are those whom you instantly connection with. The bond you share can be just as strong as a the blood-family bond. Seven generations of blood bring affection and strength that can help the patient get better and to feel more confident.

The seven generations that surround this client's life, I am able to see energies and signs moving alongside the individuals who make up the seven-generation group. Although what's happening is visible to me, it's not something I be able to see, it's not private and I don't understand what's going on. It could be a group of people talking about, singing, chanting offering prayers, or anything which is so incredible that I don't be able to comprehend. It's not my intention to participate in this.

At times, the seven generations of the family would assist on the team of warriors and also on the team of love. Though their presence was acknowledged but it was far too loud for me to effectively assist. I requested the seven generations to decide if it was okay for them to have their own section. To date, I haven't received a response from the seven generations. I'm not sure the method of contacting each seven-generation, but I can tell that everything seems to be operating. It seems like there's an energy exchange. Also, I believe that it's instantly available for all groups at the same at a time.

Once the seven generations are completed, it's time to express gratitude to all those that was involved. The process usually takes place very fast. When I first began the process, it seemed like a good moment to express my gratitude to everyone that helped. Then it's one second. The way time is working seems to be different within Quantum Room. Quantum Room. It is possible that I am making the most of my period of time with each participant however I am unable to comprehend it in the same speed while it's happening.

Chapter 4: Observer Effect

The amount of success I've had helping animals and humans has been awe-inspiring. I've asked myself many times what the reason. What is the reason this has been such a success? How come the results are happening quickly? What is the reason why results look too fantastic to be real?

The answer I have to these questions lies in the fact that these animals and people were sent to me by the universe for reasons. The universe knew those animals and humans had a problem and could I aid them. I'm not certain whether I'm able to help everyone. I'm not quite sure if it is appropriate that I'm supposed to help everyone. It's not clear if it's permitted to assist everyone. It's true that I enjoy helping those animals and the people which I am drawn by.

After and during an appointment, I'm extremely confident that what I've completed is efficient. People and animals I'm supposed help have been open to my efforts and are healing. Sometimes, I want to help but I'm not able to connect with the person. The Quantum Room could be empty or even doze off when I try to communicate with the person. I'm not sure what is work that goes on behind the scenes that is happening in the Universe. I'm thinking that I'm supposed be assisting certain people, animal or community members and they are directed at me.

There are other times where I've tried to assist someone else, but do not get the result I want. Initially, I saw this as failure. The thing I've learned is that there exists an effect known as"the observer effect. The observer effect occurs in both physics and psychology. The observer effect in psychology is the result of observed and are aware that they're being observed, they are more likely to behave in a different way. For all you non-hand washers do you have a higher likelihood to clean your hands in the restroom when you're on your own or within the company of others? The observer effect in physics indicates that electrons, particles and other particle types are also able to exhibit the characteristics of particles as well as characteristics that are characteristic of waves. In looking through Quantum Room sessions I believed were unsuccessful, I have now realized that there was improvement, even in the absence of my desired outcome I was hoping for. Examples of this include:

* The cancer will not completely disappear from the patient, but their life quality or their understanding of the situation improves

* A client dies and his family members are more able to heal faster and with less grief, and have peaceful

If you make the intention of helping the client, you'll aid the person. Although the result might not appear immediately, but it will show improvement within the lives of the person who is helping them or their family.

Two instances have occurred in which I've had a client that stated they needed help however, they really weren't. The second one is described in my book. Both individuals did get better in a short period of time; however they weren't willing to alter. When a trauma is an integral element of a person's identity is that they can't be able to let it go regardless of whether it could result in them losing their lives. I'd like to understand what the reason is but maybe in the future I'll be in a position to.

While I considered the book I was writing I was not sure if to add some events that took place within Quantum Room. Quantum Room. Would anyone believe me? Do people believe I'm more bizarre and crazy than they did? Could I be laughed of? Was I branded as a fraud? This and numerous other questions kept me awake for several months. Then I came to the conclusion that my experience was valid in my view and decided to share them with you. I truly hope that the stories that you're about to read are a good fit for you.

Sick Puppy

My friend had puppies with an acute stomach problem. The Veterinarian carried out an operation on the puppy but he wasn't reacting. I read on social media a post that said he'd made the decision to send the dog back to the vet to be put into a slumber due to declining health and discomfort. My friend asked me to delay the visit by an hour while letting me attempt to assist.

The whole Warrior team gathered. The dogs were very energetic and eager to assist. Desi was able to sniff around the puppy, and then pulled the look of an untidy string out of the stomach of the puppy. When she had pulled it around six inches then she stopped, and dipped her nose in the puppy's stomach. Within the Quantum Room Desi can be found to enter the bodies of people as well as animals. At times, she appears as if she's digging. Other times she just leans her body or head towards the person. It's like she's moving through an invisibly closed body. I could feel Desi turning her head and she thought to me that she had to loosen the string, so her puppy will be fine. Desi backed out with the opposite side of her string.

The puppy was instantly happier. He appeared to be smiley!!

The dogs from the Warrior Team moved in and began licking the puppy's entire body. After they had licked the puppy they began rubbing with the dog. It's common to see cats doing this similar thing all the time. Cats, house cats, and the tigers in TV, rub as if they are an entire family uniting.

The outside was burned the string to let the team of love to heal the string. The love team grew stronger and fed the string, it transformed into a liquid-like substance that dissolved and then flowed off.

I'm not sure what this string represents. I'm not sure what the liquid was representing. It was evident that it was content to be the liquid, and it was eager to go on with its life as the string.

In the afternoon, when I was browsing through my social media accounts, I came across a friend who was posting a story regarding the puppy. The moment he set out to bring him to the vet to be placed down the puppy was to move around and became thirsty and hungry. He hadn't had a meal in more than a day, and was hungry.

The dog was in excellent condition in only a few days! It happened in 2017, and four years on, the puppy is an extremely happy dog who is loved by all the family.

My friend hasn't mentioned the issue to me. This is like the part I played in the dog's healing disappeared from my memory, or occurred in a different dimension or reality. This happens frequently. A single person from my clients I've worked with has stated that I were able to work. It's not clear what's causing this but I've lost my self-esteem and been working on humility. It's a blessing. It's not something I'd want or require. credit.

Lady has a variety of health concerns

Working with individuals in the Quantum Room I'm often struck by the feeling that it difficult to connect with the others, as if I was watching an MLB game in the first row. I'm there, I'm there, but there's a gap. However, in this instance the person walked into my presence and gave me the most warm hug. It was longer than normal hugs as I believed that the additional connection was required to this individual. After we ended our hug glanced at her and said I was happy for her and she'd be fine.

The Quantum Room, everything is in free flow. Nothing is scheduled, and what is required to occur will take place. I don't know the reason this patient wanted to be told that she was appreciated. I don't know the reason I felt the need to share this message. A lot of things happening within Quantum Room Quantum Room are unexpected. The session was completely unexpected. Could it be that she's part of my soul group, and I did not know until I had the conversation? It's possible that I will never know an answer to this.

Desi shifts to the left rib of the client and starts digging out a stick, Hammer, as well as an empty beer bottle. We don't remove the objects, but the love team transmits the energy of love to the items. The items begin to shine, but gradually fade and fade away.

Desi Then she pulls tiny green creatures from every breast. The monsters are small and green and have large claws on their hands. They're very pissy and brutal. Like the other items, there's nothing to debride, only the energy of love. It's the same for the animals that were present in the initial items. It's just an incessant disappearance until there's nothing left.

Desi begins pulling a cable out of the bottom of the rear of the neck. Once she has gotten about a foot of cable pulled out of her back then the Martian warrior is able to take the cable away and keeps pulling. The Martian warrior gets 20 feet of cable as the turtle jumps over and begins to take away several hundred feet of cables. When the final inch of cable is cut an enormous storm roars through the back of the client and swiftly overflows with water in the Quantum Room. The storm is massive enough that it is bigger than the turtle. The storm is several hundred times larger than the gigantic turtle. The boiling clouds are forming through the storm. Numerous lightning sets are exploding around the interior of the storm. The cable is reattached the storm, and is now packed with electricity and sparks. Energy.

The love team as well as the horses and cats from the warrior team are growing to an enormous size. They're now larger than the storm, and are surrounded by the storm. They channel love energy on the storm. Huge quantities of love flow onto the rough terrain. The team slowly and the storm begin to shrink. When the storm shrinks, it transforms into a dark grey colour, lighter grey to white and finally an almost lighter pink.

The storm starts to form. It continues to expand and then transforms into what appears as the pink Himalayan salt. The salt is broken into small pieces. are tossed away by the storm until the storm ceases to is present and a few piles of salt can be seen lying on the floor of the Quantum Room. Salt begins to emit an energy I only call beautiful. The energy shifts from light pink, to pure white. The salt changes to white before disappearing.

Everyone on the Love and warrior teams are surrounded by the client with huge affection. The client experienced a shift that every member of the team and myself experienced. The patient was recovering back to normal and regaining her health. She took her breath slowly and relaxed her body and released all the tension and toxins that she was in.

She was at peace, she was recovering.

Chapter 5: Troubled Home

I was asked by a homeowner to help the homeowner to prepare a basement that would be rented to tenants. A previous tenant had lost his life to sickness and had spoken about experiencing discomfort and feeling as if the house was watching him.

The procedure was similar for animals or humans. I brought my home to the Quantum Room and enlisted the members of my warrior group to join me. The first time, none of the group members took part. In the course of reflecting over the course of several days, I came to the idea "Only that you would be required. You were the only one who could leave".

What I saw inside the basement was fascinating. Near the bottom of the stairs were three figures that I'm calling"the Watching Man. Other people refer to him as Hat Man and Shadow Man. The Watching Man typically stands around 6 feet tall and has an impressive body. It's obvious that he is a man, however, you don't know it. He is reportedly wearing a long duster coat as well as a hat or a helmet. The colors range between charcoal grey and dark black/blue. From my observations, these beings are just watching. There has never been a feeling that I was at risk when I've seen them. What I sense from these creatures is that they're interested. This is the first occasion I've witnessed more than one of the entities in one go.

I'm convinced that I'm drawn to places where I'm needed. The room was very pulsing. desire to move to the rear bedroom, in which the former tenant had been sleeping. It was a six-foot wide hole which was joined to the conduit that was flexible. Many times while working within Quantum Room, Quantum Room I find conduits connected to animals and people.

The conduit draws energies of either the animal or animal that it is connected to. They are weaker vulnerable to illness and anxiety.

The length of the conduit was extensive. It could be hundreds, thousands or millions in length. Another idea about this pipe was that it might have been an inter-dimensional portal that crossed over into another dimension. It appeared to have an infinity length to me however; it could be just a few inches in thickness and connected to an additional dimension.

It was an intense sense of anxiety and pain that was radiating out from the entrance. It's impossible for me to imagine how I could have ever slept in the room. I'm not even sure why the renter lasted for as long. I utilized my power to cut through the entry point to the conduit. After I was able to feel the link was broken and I felt my energy redirected through the conduit.

The intention of the energy was to spread love and restore. The energy was transformed in the atmosphere of the space. Once a place of pain and anxiety was now tranquility and recuperation. Healing was taking place!

When I continued to pump force into the conduit, it started to shrink. The conduit shrank from 6-foot diameter to a smaller than one foot. As I realized the conduit wouldn't fully close the conduit, I made the decision that it should to be connected so that the same thing would not occur once more. I was able fold the ends of the conduit as one would fold an tube. Once it had been turned back on itself I altered the direction of my efforts to seal and glue the pipe's end. After the conduit had been sealed it began to disappear until I was unable to be able to see it.

The hole was not completely sealed within the wall, which needed to be sealed. In the end, I applied my strength using a shielding and sealing purpose. I was looking to ensure that my home was secure in case the conduit ever came again. Once the hole was been filled with my energies, I created an energy bubble that was protective over the entire house.

In the course of closing the conduit, Three Watching Men continued to observe me.

I checked the rest of the basement but could discover no issues. To be certain I filled the whole basement with healing energy.

The Three Watching Men were now standing on the bottom of the steps. I was about to go and I didn't know what to do. I sat down for a breath, and then walked towards them. They left my way in an strange fashion. It appeared as if the three of them were the swinging gate. They swung off from the top of the stairs and didn't attempt to prevent me from doing so. It seems that I received the approval of them.

The basement has not had any further concerns with the basement at the house.

Nightmares

In most cases, I need permission prior to engaging with a client. If it's an animal the owner would have to allow me to work. In the case of child, parents will have to grant me permission. One of the only instances I've helped clients without permission was when they're in a in a coma or have emerged from an involuntary coma, but have not gained enough awareness to talk.

The patient has been admitted and taken removed from the ICU and was placed in a variety of chemically-induced sleep comas. Though she was conscious, she'd frequently complained of having nightmares of robots trying to make her the form of a machine. If you've had the privilege of being in the ICU you will know the horror she experienced. One of my friends asked to help. I obliged, even though did not have permission from her.

She walked into her Quantum Room laying down on the bed in the hospital, and many of the IV tree also followed her. It was an enormous edifice in the air above her head. It seemed like a massive twister that was coming from every direction, it was an absolute mess. I requested the warriors to aid her. All team members rushed out. Instead of Desi searching for companions every dog and cats dived into the raging chaos. In a matter of seconds, the animals began to appear with a variety of companions.

A lot of companions were taken by the super tornado! A distorted Racoon as well as a straw the blanket, tire as well as a book, a massive grasshopper and the long tube of a tire were all taken away. Animals would not leave their companions and they were determined to make it close to the removal.

Each time, the animals would spit their companions out, while the turtle and me used the power to cleanse their companions. After they had all been cleansed and sane, the team of love moved inside to heal, expand and free the companions.

The racoon appeared to shine before changing into a tiny boy who turned to me smiled, then ran off.

It appeared as if it was melting, but it morphed as a spider-like creature which sank its legs in the earth like it was roots. The creature was not moving and seemed content at the same spot.

The tire was as a tire, but bigger and balloon-like. It was the first time the tire's companion did not change to something different during the entire process.

The book caught the flame and then exploded into a bubble which then disintegrated. It was like the bubble of soap, but it could alter direction on its own. it was not encased in the air flow.

The massive grasshopper began to smile after the positive energy struck it. The back legs of two were sunk and turned into grass. Front legs were ripped away and formed a tiny fence surrounding the grass. The body then melted into the grass, and a tiny house was built there. The yard and the house weren't there for more than an instant before they were removed.

The tube seemed to be writhing around as if it was hurting as the love began flowing in the. In a matter of seconds it stopped and appeared to embrace the love energy.

With more love flowing through it, the tube transformed into something that resembled an alligator, with a bizarre lower jaw which moved along the floor like it was trying to grab things.

In the future, I would like to grasp the significance of the characters and also what they represent in their change. It doesn't seem to be a matter of appearance. Everyone started with an optimistic intention even if they look like an animal.

They begin to want to aid. They could have been with us from the age of the age of five. Many times, companions are taught behavior that helps us stay in a safe place or leads us to more positive things. One of them may start in the form of a belief that we must keep quiet in classes and refrain from speaking up because they were laughed at or ridiculed. The learned habits may hinder us in our development and growth at school or in business. They are the thoughts of those who are manifesting into the shapes I can see within the Quantum Room. In order to be precise, there's neither a real gremlin nor tire within a person. The company members appear as unpredictable appearances within the quantum space.

Haunted House

An investigation group from paranormal investigations asked me to be part of their team to clean a home. A lovely lady was experiencing issues with an entity that was in her house. The entity would shut the lights off in her bathroom while she was showering. The entity would also rub her when she was showering. The creature would appear on the other side of her bed and smack her. The creature would also walk throughout the attic. If she was asleep, it would hit her head and then hit her head.

You can imagine her being scared to fall asleep. She was scared to go back at home.

In The Quantum Room, I brought the house of her friend to my room in order to determine what caused the issue. One of the first things I discovered seemed to be a middle aged male. The man did not appear to be in contact with the female. He seemed to be going on about his work and occasionally interact with her which seemed to cause confusion in the same way it puzzled her. There were many places within her home that she'd be cold or uncomfortable were the places where they came into contact. These areas are what I would call as a "weakness" between dimensions or reality. All of the weak spots were light blue and was easy to discern.

In my gut, I realized that I must strengthen these areas in order to assist both men and women to stop the tense relationships. The areas I was focusing on were quite simple to restore. I devoted my attention to the breech area and allowed it to fill in the areas that were weak. After the tint of light blue was gone completely I realized that I was able to move onto the next gap and fix the damage.

The most beautiful reaction occurred after the last slit was closed. The lady that we helped and the man in middle age took the time to breathe deeply, then let it go. it, and smiled. It was obvious that this particular part of the issue she was experiencing was resolved.

What I came across next was an odd gremlin-like creature. It was approximately four feet tall, had gray/green in color. It was without hair and had nothing but a t-shirt. Strangely, the creature wasn't conscious of me when I was working alongside a middle-aged man. When my attention was focused upon the gremlin its focus was on myself as well. The creature charged immediately and was dispelled once it came into contact with my energy which was circling my body. The reaction was astonished and furious for the beast. It attempted to physically harm me three times more before it fled into the attic. It began throwing a massive screaming fit. It was in that same area within the attic where the woman said she'd be able to hear footsteps stomping about.

I figured it was better to let the creature let go of its energy before attempting to work with it.

When I began to search through the home to find other potential issues I noticed strings tacked to different places within the house. The kitchen, the front room, bedroom, as well as bathrooms were all connected to the walls, floor and furniture. I made use of my strength to cut off the link with the house. While the strings were cut off it appeared like they were moving by the gentle breeze. They then appeared to disappear. I'm unsure of what these strings were or the purpose for which they served but they did give me a feeling that they had to be taken away.

The grinning creature's fury had stopped, and I headed to the attic to find out the situation. It had an armchair and a tiny table. In the back of the chair was a rotating disk about five feet long.

The gremlin saw me, it (I'm not sure of the sex of the creature however it did feel as if it was a) was able to jump at the disk, then disappeared. I decided to look into the disk. I was fascinated by the nature of it and the way it functioned. It seemed like it was floating without attachments or bracings, there were no legs, and nothing to secure it I could discern. There was an electrical sensation to it. It was like an electromagnetic radiating from it.

The chair was lifted up and I slid its legs down into the disk. It appeared that the legs disappeared. As I walked through the disc when I held the chair the legs were not discernible in the background of the disk. I then decided that the best method I had in mind was to put the chair into the disk to see what happens.

In some instances, when I'm in my Quantum Room I forget that my power is much stronger than when I am inside our reality or dimension. The chair flew over the disk, as if it was connected to the rocket. A loud explosion emanated from the disk. However there was nothing. After about a minute, there was no additional activity, I concluded that the disk required to be brought back into contact to the chair. The chair slid through the disk with less force and there was a lesser amount of disturbance that was caused by the an impact.

In general, I do not engage in violence during the Quantum Room. Somehow, this animal inspired me to become in a violent way in the face of it. It seems like this violent behavior doesn't fit in to the job I'd like to achieve and so I trying to change it.

The disk appeared to serve as a gateway to the creature known as the gremlin I was aware I'd need to eliminate the disk. I wasn't sure of what I could do to solve this issue. I had a goal in mind to make the disk go away and never be able to return. I focused my mind to the disk for a number of minutes. The energy began to flow out of my fingers and then towards the disk. The disk was surrounded by energy for a couple of seconds before it went away.

When I went through the remainder of the house I felt confident that there was nothing inside the property that would make her nervous.

When I was reminiscing with the lady who was the owner of the house about what I discovered, she mentioned something which surprised me. "Thanks, the house feels good and should feel good for a couple days until the gremlin creature comes back."

The thought lingered in her thoughts for weeks. Was she thinking that? What would she do to know the creature was returning? In the process of asking the same question over and over it occurred to me that a different thought came into my mind Did she really want the Gremlin to make a be back? The answer I got was Yes. I'm not sure what the reasons are, but I think that she wanted the item to be returned.

After a few months of my first trip to the residence I returned in The Quantum Room to see if the creature that was a gremlin had returned. Indeed, it had returned. As soon as the creature noticed my return the creature began to run through the house in a frantic attempt to escape me. I chased it until the attic, where it vanished. The disk wasn't located in the attic. I'm not quite sure what the creature did to get off from me.

The truth is that I squandered this chance horribly. I treated the creature as a threat, and not as a creature which might have required my assistance. I was tempted to harm it since it hurt an innocent woman. I made a mistake. I'll continue looking for the gremlin and try to help it in any way I could.

Chapter 6: What Exactly Is Energy Healing?

The practice of energy healing (or Reiki in certain areas) is an alternative therapy in which people utilize their hands to transmit the energies of the universe between the practitioner and the patient.

If you're interested in what it is, then energy healing is believed to tap the energetic fields that surround the body, using their hands to act as instruments for therapy. Reiki is derived from the Japanese word'rei' (universal) and 'ki' (mysterious environment) (life energy). It is a method to provide your body and soul with the energies of the cosmic sphere.

According to healers of the energy field, can easily stay in your body when there is psychological or physical stress. It usually results in an adverse effect on both our mental and physical wellbeing, which is why we'd prefer to rid ourselves of it to restore balance in the body.

If you've experienced the practice of acupuncture, it's an alternative that isn't as invasive! Energy therapy, which seeks to restore energy flow throughout the body is fantastic to help relax, reduce discomfort, speeding up your body's healing process and much more.

Energy Medicine can unlock energy in your life, which can bring energy, resilience, joy and awe - aswell with increased vigor for your mind, body, as well as your spirit! The balance of your energy helps regulate your body's chemical balance and regulate your hormones. You'll have better mood, and even be more productive. Energy Medicine is called the self-care and advancement path for the coming years however it allows people to now adapt and excel in the current challenges of the 21st century.

How Is Energy Medicine Used?

Energy medicine practices can be seen in a wide range of healing practices and cultures. These are now being used at hospitals for a non-invasive procedure that can increase the standard of care and complement Western medical professionals' efforts. The intention behind these treatments is to restore imbalances in energy fields believed to exist within and surrounding the human body.

The common reason for mood disorders is to seek out energy medicine treatments (anxiety or depressive).

"I'm out of sorts...

* Hyperactivity or sleepiness.

* Constant ache.

* Cancer.

* Stress-related illnesses.

* Fatigue.

* Recovering from a surgery.

Here are the top popular methods of energy healing:

Reiki Energy Healing

Reiki originates from two Japanese words: 'Rei' meaning God's wisdom and 'Ki that means energy. This type of therapy is utilized alongside traditional medicines for treating illnesses. "Ki," or energy, is utilized to aid others during this form of therapy. Numerous hand movements as well as specific symbols are employed to tap into the power of the universe for healing the body.

Reiki helps with headaches, colds, flu as well as stomachaches. Pranic Healing is efficient in the treatment of serious illness like heart diseases.

Pranic healing is about harnessing the life force within your body to repair the energy of the body. This therapy focuses on an individual's energy, or aura. The energy is used to eliminate any toxins that are in the body thus speeding the healing process for physical ailments.

Crystal Healing

This therapeutic approach uses crystals and stones are used to remove toxins out of the body. Crystals and stones can are able to have different impacts on your body, and can address emotional, physical and spiritual problems. They remove negative energy from the body, which can cause physical and mental pain.

Quantum Healing

Quantum healing is based upon the concepts of harmony and pleasure. Breathing and visualizing energies increase levels of energy within the body. Quantum

Healing is not only spiritual but is also a positive influence on the immune system.

Qigong

In order to restore the body's equilibrium, the qigong treatment practiced. Qigong is a tradition that dates back to 4,000 years and involves synchronized bodily breathing, movements and meditation in order to improve wellbeing as well as spirituality. It is an ancient form of Chinese traditional medicine. It is thought to restore the health of your body's positive energy. This is necessary to maintain a healthy body.

Energy Medicine believes that energy is an active, real-time and moving element that affects numerous aspects of health as well as satisfaction. It is believed that in Energy Medicine, energy is the drug, but energy also serves as the patient. The body is repaired by activating the body's natural healing powers; also, you help the body heal itself by returning energy that has become unbalanced, weak or off balance.

Energy Medicine is both a complement to the existing treatments for medical conditions and also a complete system of care and assistance for self. It could assist in treating physical ailments and emotional as well as mental illness, and may also help to promote higher levels of well-being and optimal efficiency.

These are the basic concepts of energy medicine:

Energy--both subtle and electromagnetic energy--help to build the energetic system of the physical body.

The overall health of these energy sources, in terms of flow equilibrium, and harmony -- is seen by the well-being of our bodies.

To beat illness and maintain a healthy body your body's vitality should:

You must move and you should have room for movement. Energies can become blocked due to pollutant and muscle, or any other limitation as well as chronic stress the interference of other energies.

They move in patterns that are predictable. These patterns usually align with the physical structure and the functions they are able to sustain and animate. The flow process is the result of function.

From the smallest level of DNA double helix up to the macro level, where both sides of the brain is responsible for both sides of our body. Likewise, the right side is in control of the left side of the body.

Keep a healthy balance with the other energy sources -- Energies can be unable to maintain their balance naturally due to prolonged tension or other causes which keep specific energy systems functioning in a state of survival.

• Non-invasively maintain and repair the flow, balance and harmony in the energy system using:

The act of tapping, rubbing or twisting or rubbing specific energy points of the skin.

Hands that are whirling across the skin in certain energy paths.

A posture or exercise designed to give a specific effect on energy.

Focused use of the mind to change certain energies. A region that is surrounded by healing energy (one person's energies influence another)

Chapter 7: The Basic Energy Systems

The energy structure is just complex and intricate as the physical structure. Though I've been conscious of the energetic body and their roles, the significance of each system came to light when I started helping others in their healing. It also became apparent that each of these systems is acknowledged and discussed within at least one other cultural traditional healing practices. Certain systems, such as the chakras, meridians and the aura, are widely known. Others haven't been as well-known.

Eden Energy Medicine addresses the 9 energy systems that are the most important every day:

* Meridians, Chakras, Aura, and the Basic Grid.

* The Celtic Weave.

* The Five Rhythms.

* Three-way Warmer.

* Electrics and Radiant Circuits.

Meridians are energy conduits which serve as the body's main bloodstream of energy. Each meridian flows across the surface of skin, in the area where it can be the most susceptible to being impacted and then deep inside the body. It is able to transfer energy to some organs, or biological system. Meridians connect body, mind as well as the soul.

The 14 meridians consist by 12 connected segments (typically named for one of the major organs they manage) and two lines of energy that are known as Central and the Governing. The 12 meridians are joined into a single canal that supplies vitality to muscles, organs and cells. For me, the meridians appear to be like a web of flowing ribbons in rainbow colors that flow across the body.

Chakras The seven main chakras that are located in the spinal column (other minor chakras can be located in the entire body). The chakras function as energy discs, or pools of energy which cleanse and nourish the organs that are located near them.

They control the endocrine system, and also store data about an individual's life. Emotional, mental, physical as well as spiritual events can also be encoded and processed. Every major chakra is comprised of seven levels. The deepest that extends to the Grid of Basic and those that are the most outermost are in touch with the aura.

Aura The aura similar to the atmosphere of Earth, encompasses and covers the body. It's the body's outermost energetic system made up of seven levels, or nested field of auric energy (think Russian dolls) with seven bands that run from the bottom up to the highest. Each band or layer has an important function, but the overall function of the aura is:

* Filter to shield the body from harm or destructive energies.

* An antenna designed to draw positive energy.

The aura is responsible for processing the required elements from the surrounding environment like sunlight, as well as assists in keeping the magnetic field. Aura's proper functioning can have profound effects on the physical, emotional as well as spiritual health.

It is the Fundamental Grid: A matrix or grid pattern is a part of the body. all over the body. It forms the foundation of other systems of energy and is the energy source of the entire body. It's slow and dense. It is slow and dense. Grid is the primary structure for our energy systems, similar to what the skeletal system provides for our bodies. Additionally, it provides instant support to bones. It is impossible for people to fully thrive when the Grid is damaged, and may have a difficult time getting their energy back or fully recuperating, physically as well as emotionally. Every aspect of our body's energy is supported when the Grid is in good health and strong.

Celtic Weave: This energy system is similar to the weaving of a material or a basket. It helps in the making of the perfect container for all the body's energy. It also functions as a connective tissues throughout your body's energy. While meridians are similar to the streams of water and chakras are similar to pools The Celtic weave is an internet.

It joins all our energy systems to form an interconnected system of communication via the crisscrossing of large and small figure 8s along with various geometric patterns. The patterns that cross the Celtic Weave are a representation of the fundamental forms seen in the natural world. It is believed that the Celtic Weave will be increasingly apparent as your body's energy and the overall health increase. Affirming the healing process with a strengthening of the Celtic Weave can be a good option. This will help to secure the gains.

The Rhythms: A complicated series of pulses referred to by The Five Elements, Five Seasons or Five Rhythms moves through all of the bodies energy. They are the fundamental energy patterns which flow through the body and are imprinted the energy systems of all other bodies.

The model is based on the tradition-based Chinese medical practices The Five Rhythm Model depicts the beat of life's rhythms that shapes our human experiences and cycles. Each meridian pulsates according to one of five Elements or Rhythms and are represented through symbols like the metaphors of Water and Wood, as well as Fire, Earth, and Metal.

The Five Rhythms give a framework to recognize and address problems with chronic health, bad behavior patterns, as well as emotional problems. Triple Warmer can be described as a meridian or it is a Radiant Circuit, but it is also able to perform a variety of other purposes that I often use the term "a completely different energy system. It regulates the immune system, the fight-flight-or-freeze response, and the body's survival behaviors in particular.

Triple Warmer energy is a direction of travel, however the energy flow is extremely fluctuating. It is moving with a heavy slow, sluggish motion sometimes, and then massive bursts of intense force at other. Triple Warmer appears reddish brown to me a lot times, but it does have the appearance of a yellow flash during moments of intense bursts.

In the form of it is a Radiant Circuit Its energies can be distributed throughout the body. It is able to draw energies from any meridians within the body (save that of the Heart) when it needs it. The individual is able to switch into autopilot mode to perform normal activities since it's the one who controls the body's routines. It is also an intermediary, directing your immune system to know what it should accept and which to avoid or not accept.

Circuits Radiant in the traditional Chinese healing The Radiant Circuits (also called the Strange Flows or Extraordinary Vessels) are subtle flows of energy which help and support the other systems of energy including the meridians. They nourish pleasure and other positive sensations due to the fact that they have a high sensitivity to thoughts and feelings. The stimulation of the Radiant Circuits could stimulate both the inner joy as well as the Inner Physician, that will in turn heal and harmony.

Radiant Circuits are older (in terms of the development) than meridians. They do not have a limit on routes. They instead move swiftly wherever they're needed radiating radiant light that draws vital energy from the surroundings and triggers healing within the body.

The Electricians The Electrics along with the Celtic Weave as well as the Five Rhythms are an energy system that influences the other energy systems. The reason for this is that the Electrics comprise of the electrical components of other energy systems ranging from the Aura up to the Basic Grid.

On an electrical level electricity helps bring charge to cells and connect them organs, cells, and energy systems. In addition, they influence and are influenced through the nervous system and the heart. Electrical energy is the most dense and most easily quantifiable of all the energy that our bodies produce.

Chapter 8: The Energy Medicine Pillars

Though conventional theories cannot be able to explain the occurrences that occur and the various irregularities that highlight weaknesses in a model and contribute to its enhancement. The only explanation available for the data on heart transplants can be more rational than the heart is a magnet (in actual fact, the electric field that the heart has is 60 times more powerful than the brain and the magnetic field of the heart is at times 500 times more powerful, as per some estimations) and this field is a source of information regarding the individual.

* Reach

Energy medicine is able to be a significant influence on the whole spectrum of physical ailments since it addresses bodily processes from their root energy levels. Energy medicine focuses on the energetics that are surrounded, penetrated, and help support body functioning and structure (e.g. organs, cells and blood vessels, lymph) (e.g. the immune system respiratory as well as cardiovascular). The expression of genes is also affected by technology for energy therapy.

Energy flow can be resolved through tapping, holding or rubbing certain spots of energy which can trigger changes in the course of the disease as opposed to the symptom-relief that is typical of multiple sclerosis treatment.

* Efficiency

Energy medicine regulates biological processes with precise accuracy as well as speed and flexibility. Treatments for energy medicine target the causes of particular illnesses and systems and provide information thousands of times faster than chemical signals. They also offer rapid feedback to physicians which allows therapies to be adjusted for best results.

Balance and strengthening the energetics which surround and circulate through the heart of a post-coronary person creates an inner environment that aids in the healing process and restores.

* Practicality

Energy medicine helps to heal and prevents sickness by using methods that are inexpensive, simple and minimally invasive. Energy medicine uses precise movements that are accompanied by postures, techniques that are hands-on, do not require high-tech equipment, and will not trigger unexpected reactions. Examining any disruptions to an individual's flow of energy through kidneys can lead to treatments which are more adaptable and precise than medical or surgery. It can be used to prevent the risk of harm to an organ.

* Patient Empowerment

The practice of energy medicine is based on self-help techniques that can be employed in the home setting, promoting an increased patient-practor relationship during the process of healing. The self-administered methods of energy medicine can help to detect imbalances within mechanisms, perform remedial actions to build strong energetic patterns in the body. Patients with cirrhosis can use techniques frequently to control the energetic imbalances which impact the liver, and increase its ability to heal.

* Quantum Compatibility

Remote healers, therapeutic impact of prayer and the role of intention for healing can be utilized in the field of energy medicine. Energy medicine studies the areas that alter consciousness, and operate through the passage of time (macroscopic quantum interplay) which is the basis for a hypothesis about why anticipation and desire have profound effects, as evidenced through the placebo effect as well as remote healing.

The patients suffering from cancer can be trained in techniques to tap into in the power to heal through focused intent and demonstrated how the images and thoughts they think of affect the way they recover.

* Holistic Orientation

Energy medicine encourages the integration of mind, body and soul, which results not only in a focus on healing but also increased well-being, calm and a zest for life. Energy medicine is based on the idea that the mind, body and the spirit are directly connected and their harmonious connection is encouraged.

People suffering from ulcerative colitis can learn how emotional tensions can cause symptoms, and they can receive remedies that rapidly alter the energy underlying these conflict.

In its essence, traditional medicine is focused on the biochemistry of cells organs, tissues and. The fundamental focus of energy medicine concentrates on fields that control and regulate the growth and maintenance of tissues, cells, and organs, as being strategies that influence these areas.

Energy medicine offers many advantages over traditional treatment of medicine. They could be considered the main factors that define the energy medicine field as an important improvement in health care.

Reach--energy medicine could affect the whole spectrum of physical ailments as it addresses the biological process at its energy source. Human bodies are an energy system that is living, not just the combination of its mechanical parts. The skin produces around 30 photons per square centimeter every second.

Every cell generates electromagnetic radiation. Every bodily function is governed by electrical signals. Western medicine, on contrary, tends to focus on the chemistry of the body without attention to its energy sources or organizing fields. In addition, the majority of treatments are pharmacological or surgery-related interventions instead of alternative energy therapies. Yet, recent research does oppose this asymmetric approach. The impact of energy fields in regulating gene expression could indeed lie at the root of the energy medicine's huge impact for curing and even preventing the most elusive health conditions.

The results of hundreds of scientific studies in the past 50 years have proven that invisible forces from the electromagnetic spectrum exert an impact on each level of biological regulation. Particular electromagnetic patterns influence DNA, RNA and protein synthesis. They also alter the shape and function of proteins, as well as regulate gene regulation, cell division, differentiation, and morphogenesis (the method that cells join to form the organs, tissues and even cells).

Growth of the nerve, hormones and function are the basic processes that play a an important contribution to the development of our lives.

What does this lack of respect for the role of energy in regulating biological processes mean for the future of medical practice? This leads to more intrusive treatments which are less effective in identify the causes of the disease as well as less capable of altering the mechanisms it could be influencing with precision.

As an example, when an imbalance in electromagnetic fields prompts the body to produce the chemical needed to restore balance, for instance progesterone or estrogen. The chemical is created precisely and precisely where it's needed. The energy treatments designed to boost estrogen and progesterone levels send electromagnetic signals into the body and cause it to create the necessary hormone using its body's natural system.

If drugs enter bloodstreams they are based on guesswork and averages, which is why they can travel into and interact with areas of the body which do not belong which can result, for example devastating increases in strokes, heart diseases as well as breast cancer in women who've had hormone replacement therapy. These are also known as side effects. Every year, somewhere around 100,000-300,000 individuals within the United States die from medications which are taken according to prescription, but inadvertently.

The ability of energy medicine to effectively alter the energetics that drive all biological functions by modifying the way that the biological paradigm is not able to do can is the most important pillar in its capability to overcome the shortcomings of our current health methods. Traditional medicine is unable to develop techniques that can be used to influence genes' expression levels as well as early detection of disease and prevention, as well as intervention in macro-processes like immunity because there isn't an approach to developing proactive treatments that focus on the energy fields of your body.

* Efficiency - With accuracy, speed and the ability to adapt, energy interventions can influence biological processes. For relaying data within biological systems electromagnetic frequencies can be a hundred times more effective than chemical signals like neurotransmitters or hormones as per a research study that was based on studies conducted at Oxford University in the 1970s.

A lot of body's regulator chemical substances, like hormones, move less than one centimeter per second. However, an electromagnetic wave may have covered about three-quarters the distance to the moon during this duration. The signals from acupuncture have been found to produce information several orders of magnitude quicker that nerve signals. Apart from the exponentially higher rate of energy intervention however, the vast majority of data transmitted by chemical diffusion goes to waste since that a large portion of the process involves the creation and breaking of bonds between chemicals. Physical chemical signals are 100 times more effective and infinitely faster than energy-based transmissions.

What kind of communications do you think your trillion-celled colony would like? Do the math. Traditional medicine continues to deny the many ways that energy could transfer information within biological systems (with certain notable exceptions for instance, the usage of heart pacemakers, frequency harmonics that break down kidney stones, the use of pulsed stimulation machines, as well as using magnets in treating facial paralysis, tendonitis and atrophy of the optic nerve). However, conventional medicine has not had any difficulty embracing diagnostic tools that are based on the concept of information as energy.

MRIs, EEGs, ECGs, EMGs, and CAT scans have shown ability to detect sickness without invasive procedures by studying the frequency ranges of body's chemical tissue, organs and tissues. The characteristic electromagnetics of healthy tissues and those that are damaged can be detected in images scanned. Each tissue with disease will have its own unique electromagnetic signature, and it differs from that of healthy cells surrounding it.

Practitioners of energy medicine have already claimed to detect imbalances in energy fields of the body and then directly address them to ensure that the patterns of waveforms generated by damaged tissue or malfunctioning system are altered, and they are covered by energetic fields which have a therapeutic impact with the help mechanical equipment.

As long as these techniques can be formulated and taught, energy therapy can provide therapies that are far more precise than medications as well as more adaptable and less invasive than surgery. significantly reducing the amount of time needed for healing, while avoiding unwanted negative side consequences.

The practicality of energy medicine encourages the healing process and prevents sickness through methods that are simple affordable, non-invasive, and inexpensive. It has been known that survival is linked to the ability to identify and fix energy imbalances. Prior to consuming a new plant, tribesmen could tell whether its energy were harmful. Traditional medicine is designed to keep the body in good health through keeping the body's energy circulating and balanced.

The use of energy to move was utilized for healing in every civilization and system of medicine prior even our system. The traditional Chinese medical practices maintained the health of the body by keeping the energy fields in place to support it. Since disrupted energy causes similar disturbances to the body's physical (similar as how the energy field that is carried by the embryo of a salamander serves as a blueprint for an adult) and maintaining healthy energies is considered to be the path to a healthy lifestyle and prevention of sickness.

In fact, in many regions of the ancient China it was customary to pay the doctor when you were healthy. In the event of illness The doctor would work for hours trying to cure the patient, however you would not have to pay as the physician not kept the health of your energy system for you to stay clear of the illness.

The injection of energy can be part of the process of healing in a planned process. The primary type of energy used is called mechanical energy like the spark generated by pressing the button of a gas-grill lighter. This is due to how the force applied to certain substances can be converted into electricity. This is also known by the name piezoelectricity (derived from the Greek term piezein which refers to pressing or squeezing).

When you apply pressure to crystalline structures like bones, muscles, and collagen, a current could be generated. This can be the basis for Acupressure, acupuncture, as well as tapping or massage of energy points. Furthermore, the energy produced by the piezoelectrical process can be transmitted through connective tissue in the body. Another way that energy could be used to heal is to surround tissues with electromagnetic fields. In the event that a healer's hands, or a device that is magnetic are applied to a specific area or body part, energy inside the tissue is returned to its proper the proper alignment and balance according to theory at the very least.

Another option is to send electrical signals through the body similar to the way that cardiac pacemakers and pulsed magnetic stimulation devices are able to do. A highly speculative, but necessary method to explain anomalies, such as distant healing as well as other non-local impacts requires macro-level quantum field.

Although electrical devices magnetic, crystals and needles, scents as well as ingested medications are used in all forms of energy therapy The human hand is the tool employed by the most amount of practitioners to effectively transferring and harmonising the body's fields and energy. A lot of the techniques described in the standard manuals and books include hands-on procedures to bring back harmony and balance to the energy system of the body.

The practitioner can link specific areas of energy on the skin through applying pressure, massaging by pinching, twisting or twisting. Since all hands have an electromagnetic charge that can be detected they can be utilized to wrap around specific areas of the body, generating an electromagnetic field, or hands may be utilized to shift and align body energies by following specific energy paths across the skin.

Some other non-invasive, easily accessible methods include the use of certain postures or movements to help to improve the health of the body's energy systems. These non-invasive treatments are frequently considered in healthcare environments, in line with the belief that the least intrusive approach that is most likely to improve the condition is to be employed initially.

They aren't just readily accessible and can be integrated into the doctor's range with some continuous education. But their supposed anti-invasive and non-invasive properties suggest that they could also prove extremely cost-effective compared with conventional medical practices' rapidly increasing cost and adverse economic effects.

* Patient Empowerment Self-help methods in energy medicine which can be utilized in the home setting, promoting an improved patient-therapist relationship during the process of healing. The term "energy" is utilized to describe two aspects of the field of energy medicine. Energy

refers to both the medication as well as the patient.

The body is healed by activating the body's inherent healing powers (energy to treat) as well as by reinforcing energies which are fragile, disorganized or unbalanced (energy as a patient). The patient may be provided with various exercises or positions that are designed to create particular energy-related effects, that are both positive and negative. The self-administration of strategies can help them to stimulate their inner healer as well as provide balance to particular energy systems that require attention.

The energy medicine is typically administered within three different settings:

• As an all-in-one solution to deal with physical problems.

* To complement different approaches to medical care.

As part of a set of self-care and self help practices People can learn to recognize the signs that certain vital energy systems are not in equilibrium, and then perform corrective procedures and create strong energy patterns that aid in illness prevention using the energy medicine method as a self-care approach.

Although conventional medicine might suggest exercise, healthy diet, stress-reduction and other sensible ways to enhance overall health, its primary treatments consist of radiation, medicine, and surgeries and all require the intervention of an expert in health care. Energy medicine, on contrary, recognizes the energy field as a constantly moving force within every human being and can be administered by self. This is a democratic practice by definition. All people are born with the capacity to recover their own bodies. Energy medicine can teach people how make use of these energy sources to treat illness and improve their overall health.

* Quantum Compatibility--Energy medicine employs non-linear notions congruent with remote healing, prayer's therapeutic influence, and the function of purpose in healing. This topic was discussed in the past. The biggest flaw within Western medical practice is that the fundamental paradigm is centuries further behind the current state of physical science. Einstein's revolutionary formula for demonstrating that energy can be interchangeable with matter was released in 1905.

This discovery revealed, much more than just a technicality in science the fact the fact that Newtonian Physics, which focuses on the mechanisms of living only provides an insight into the larger story. In 1945, on August 6 1945, the legend of Prometheus that stole fire from gods, was transformed into the terrifying mythological issue of a naive humanity being capable of eliminate itself. The realization that the billiard ball-like particles that were a century ago composed of tiny particles of energy, each with its unique pattern of negative and positive charges, spin rate and frequency pattern -- is about changing the way we think about the most beloved Promethean innovations, including mobile phones, televisions and computers. They are all founded upon electromagnetic interactions.

Scientists gain insight into nature's tiny parts of the structure, including baryons, quarks, and mesons, there is speculation that matter is not made up of any particle at all and instead comprises string of energy that vibrates. Physical bodies are constantly moving and vibrating in response to the various energies in the environment.

Although a few treatments in Western medicine are founded on the premise that energy forms the heart of or at least tightly connected with physical matter researchers from a variety of disciplines work within this framework. For instance, they are taking note of the possible explanation force of field theories that have been neglected in their capacity to store and carry information, have quantum characteristics like impacts that are not local, and also connect with the mind, they are distinct from the ones we have currently. Even though nature's powerful and weak quantum forces are thought to exert their effects only on subatomic levels theories of fields have been created that operate on biological systems are carried out at a distance via the macroscopic quantum interaction.

This could be the reason some of the well-documented and widely observed positive effects of prayer on health and remote healing and also the role of the intention process or placebo effects, as well as the other psychological components that affect healing and health.

Another baffling observation that reveals an inequities of the conventional medicine paradigm, while showing a advantage of the energy medicine approach is the impact of intention and intent on the physical systems both inside and outside within the bodies of the individual who is expressing the intent. For instance following a course on how visualize to stop the breakdown of the red blood cell inside the test tube that was placed in a room that was far away the participants achieved the statistically significant result as they attempted to reduce the speed of degrading cells.

Studies that demonstrate the value of intentions in both social and physical processes range in scope from the effects of concentrated thought on the germination of seeds to massive reductions in the rate of crime following the introduction of groups of the meditators in troubled areas.

Chapter 9: Holistic Orientation

Energy medicine encourages the integration between mind, body, and the spirit. It results not only in the pursuit of healing but also improved health as well as peace and enthusiasm for living. Diagnostics and therapy have a major difference between traditional and energy medical practices. Energy medicine sees the human as a connected energy system that influences the body, the mind, as well as the spirit. Diagnosis refers to the presence of imbalances or disturbances within the body's energetic system. In particular, there's certain evidence suggesting that, when you suffer from cancer, your energy systems can be chaotic and lacking coherence. However, in the case of multiple sclerosis, they're very well-organized that they do not have flexibility. Treatment does not address the disease or symptoms as such. The purpose of treatment is to correct these imbalances in energy. Some symptoms are helpful for knowing the causes of imbalances as well as in determining whether the treatment is working However, they're not the primary focus.

Traditional medicine addresses kidney diseases by focusing on the kidney itself (leaving surgical and medication as the only alternatives) the energy medicine addresses the energy systems which affect the kidneys.

These energies aren't always only restricted to the kidneys. They tend to be systemic, being distributed throughout the body. In reality, energy therapy offers a variety of approaches which have a direct impact throughout the body. One method by that energy therapies can provide this universal effect is in the connective tissue and is believed to function as the body's communication system by many practitioners. Every body organ is contained within the organ that is the largest in the body. It functions as an electronic semiconductor made of liquid crystal capable of storing energy increasing signals, filtering information as well as moving information the same way, but not in another. The connective tissue acts as a massive electrochemical semiconductor in liquid crystals that can perform energy intervention, it is possible to be transmitted to all cells inside the body at all times.

This impact on the whole body has many advantages. In particular, as mentioned, when medications aimed to correct chemical imbalances in specific regions of the body circulate through the circulatory system and interfere with the balance of chemicals in non-targeted organs as well as systems. Energies, on contrary, get sent via connective tissues, which allows for the administration of information all over the body at simultaneously.

It allows the energy being transferred to integrate to the energy system in the body. The result is harmony in self-regulation. Negative effects that are serious from hand-on treatments for energy are really, not common and the most commonly encountered issues involving excessive energy transfer at a too rapid rate for a physically fragile person to be able to tolerate. In addition, energy treatment options allow for rapid activation of the body's signaling system that is clinically secure, according to their practitioners however, it's additionally holistic in its ability to link the mind, body and the spirit.

The impact of mind-set on overall health of your body has been extensively researched. The people who had a negative explanation style were more at likelihood of suffering from physical ailments as compared to those who had positive explanation styles as per a study of 35 years. study that was conducted over a long period of time.

The effect of cognition upon biological processes is immediately and very decisive. Concentrated intention can actually bend or break the sturdiness of DNA strands. This could lead to the possibility that DNA functions as an antenna that is which is sensitive to electromagnetic fields as well as cognitive processes that ultimately control the expression of genes.

Energy psychology and energy medicine (energy psychology is one of the subsets of energy medicine similar to psychiatry, which is a subset within conventional medicine) offer strategies to direct influence on the energetics that are associated with psycho-psychological process.

It's feasible to address emotional problems with a way that promotes good psychological health using this approach. It is a powerful and direct approach to interacting with ideas emerging from mental health and behavioral medicine.

Additionally, many of the traditional practices being revivified through energy medicine are spiritual practices along with medical processes Some practitioners even consider that the energy they generate could be the gateway into the realm of spirituality.

Furthermore, the medical system based upon the biological model must fight the biological paradigm to take in the latest findings and implications for health the importance of awareness as well as intention and subtle energy on physical systems.

Chapter 10: Energy Therapy

The energy treatments are holistic therapy techniques that focus on body, mind as well as the spirit. The term "alternative" or complementary treatment is one of the medical terms doctors use to refer to the treatments. The use of energy therapies is becoming well-known for their ability to treat a broad array of medical conditions.

Over the course of thousands of years individuals have relied on the energy healing techniques. Concepts of energy therapy are based on the notion that illness and imbalances arise from obstructions or imbalances that occur in the body's biofield that is not visible to us.

The energy treatment methods improve wellbeing and health by harmonising the energy fields inside and surrounding the body. They can also assist in the development of positive thinking and emotional states.

The treatments for energy therapy are carried out by a licensed medical professional or a healthcare practitioner using a range of non-invasive techniques.

Energy therapy is often used in conjunction with traditional therapies. It comes in many varieties. Acupressure, Reiki, and mats for acupressure are the most well-known methods of treatment for energy.

Acupressure and Reiki

Reiki is a form of treatment using energy to help heal. The doctor Dr. Mikao Usui developed the method in Japan in the 1920s. Reiki principles are based on the idea that every person has an inherent capacity to heal themselves. The Reiki practitioner is believed to be in a position to alter their clients' universal life force energy to aid in healing naturally.

The Reiki therapy involves the practitioner placing their hands close to the body of the patient. Based on the individual's needs The practitioner will usually keep the hands at a specific spot for at least three minutes. Acupressure, just like acupuncture is one of the methods used in conventional Chinese medical treatment (TCM).

In lieu of needles pressure can be used to stimulate the acupoints and allow qi or energy in the body to flow in a fluid manner. This can be accomplished by oneself or assisted by an expert.

* Acupuncture

Acupuncture is one TCM practice that involves manipulating the energy in the body. Modern medicine, on contrary, has demonstrated its effectiveness by explaining the alteration of the body that occurs as a consequence of this practice. This includes:

* Reactions to inflammation.

* Neurochemical reactions for example, the synthesis serotonin, dopamine and endorphins.

An increase in the number of immunological response, for example white blood cells count.

* Reactions to the circulatory system.

This procedure involves placing needles that are blunt in tip into areas of acupressure within the body. It helps clear stagnated or blocked Qi to help restore the balance of the body and aid in healing.

The treatment should be carried out by a qualified certified Acupuncturist who is certified and competent. They must hold an advanced master's degree or more as well as many with doctoral degrees in

Acupuncture. They are also required to be able to pass the National Certification Commission for Acupuncture and Oriental Medical's National board examination.

What's the purpose behind this therapy?

Treatments for energy are designed to improve the flow of energy. It can be used to treat a specific illness or for improving their general health, and many use it alongside other treatment. The sessions for energy therapy are typically provided in wellness and massage establishments, in addition to traditional medical facilities like clinics and hospitals.

Energy therapy is often used by patients for:

* Sleep disorders.

• Wound healing and issues with blood pressure.

* Rheumatoid arthritis.

* Depression and anxiety.

* Stress.

* Anxiety.

* Pain.

* Migraine.

* Nausea and vomiting.

* Exhaustion.

Chapter 11: Is Energy Treatment Supported By Science?

Although it's difficult to evaluate certain aspects of energy therapies, like the body's energy level, scientifically speaking, certain evidence suggests the need for the therapies for specific diseases.

Based on the results of a study that focused on energy therapy, one treatment can reduce carpal tunnel pain as well as bad feeling. Additionally, it could be beneficial to wellbeing, stress levels, and quality of sleep. The therapists conducted the 30 minute sessions in close proximity while some were using soft touch that is immobile.

The study of acupuncture, Reiki Research studies on acupuncture, Reiki and Acupressure are in the following list:

* Acupressure studies

An experiment has shown the possibility that acupressure could reduce tension and discomfort. A larger number of high-quality tests, however need to be carried out in order to verify these findings.

Researchers reached the conclusion that acupressure was a reliable cost-effective, safe and affordable non-surgical solution for chronic lower back pain.

* Reiki investigation

An article released in 2021 looked at the effectiveness of Reiki therapy, physiotherapy, as well as medication in relieving back pain, and improving the quality of life for those suffering from intervertebral disc herniation. Based on the research findings, Reiki can be a cost-effective method to reduce pain immediately and increase the quality of your daily life.

Acupuncture can help ease the fibromyalgia and migraine pain. It may also ease the low back or neck discomfort. Researchers have concluded that acupuncture is an alternative treatment option as it has a few adverse consequences and is cost-effective.

Acupuncture can also aid in:

"Hot flashes.

* Nausea.

* Cancer-related fatigue.

* Signs and symptoms of allergic to rhinitis.

* Recurring allergies symptoms.

Additionally one of the most comprehensive studies on acupuncture that included 1792 patients, showed that the treatment is effective to treat chronic pain. It is, therefore, an effective referral option.

* Outlook

A majority of patients are protected receiving energy therapies with experienced practitioners. An interested practitioner could contact them to discuss questions or discuss the treatment goals. Additionally, they can learn about the training and experiences.

Before starting any therapy new one should speak an expert in healthcare in particular if the therapy will be included in their current therapy plan. When a pregnant woman and/or taking drugs or suffers from a medical issue it is important to consider alternatives to conventional therapies, like energy therapy to determine which treatment is appropriate for their needs. The use of energy therapies should not be the sole treatment for life-threatening or severe ailments or signs

Healing Tools

From the beginning of recorded history the people of all times have relied on tools for healing. Minerals, plants and the healing properties of metals' properties made them effective tools in the arsenal of healing of shamans and healers from the past midwives, healers, and other medicine both women and men. Music has been used for healing as well, as well as modern technologies have enabled these and many other treatments more available more than ever. Jewelry, wands for healing or music instruments, as well as tuning forks are but a handful of examples of the numerous healing tools that are available.

Rudraksha malas are a type of energy-based beads believed to possess therapeutic qualities. The rudraksha tree is an Asian evergreen tree. The blossoms of the fruit can be used to make jewelry. It is believed to bring peace, focus and security to the wearer. In India Monks and Yogis consider that the rudraksha beads represent the divine essence of Shiva and is a spiritual ally.

Certain minerals contain characteristics that can be useful for healing purposes. Copper is known since the beginning of time for its therapeutic properties. Copper bracelets continue to be well-known as healing tools because of its anti-inflammatory qualities. A lot of arthritis sufferers wear copper-based jewelry and claim that it eases pain and swelling However, the use of copper to heal isn't solely due to its anti-inflammatory qualities. Consuming it internally the benefits of copper are also evident. The use of copper has been demonstrated in studies to decrease the risk of developing ulcers that are caused by anti-inflammatory medications as well as copper taken internally can heal stomach ulcers.

Copper is also an excellent conductor of energy. This makes it the ideal material to make the healing tools. A lot of people believe that wands made from mixing copper with different gemstones and crystals are effective tools for healing.

Forks for tuning are an additional beneficial instrument. Each tuning fork represents an exact note. Many people believe that hitting two forks in a row will help alter the body. Pure sound may instantly bring a sense of tranquility for certain individuals and aid people in attaining emotional balance. Forks for tuning are commonly used alongside other therapeutic methods like reiki massage, yoga, or massage.

The use of music can also serve to treat. A few artists specialize in producing music with calming properties while listening to music could provide a wide range of health benefits. Music is able to lower tension and create an atmosphere of focus. Subliminal and music messages are frequently mixed in order to attain a goal like weight loss as well as self-confidence enhancement and finding a long-term relationship partner.

Chapter 12: The way it got started

In the beginning of 2014 my wife and I prepared for a three-week vacation to Europe. I was so stressed and distracted that I did not think about the chest pains I felt during the late at night. I tried sleeping without the pain. It didn't make any difference. The pain got ever more severe and progressively stronger. It was quite unique, a move-related pain. It could happen located in one area, but the next day, in a different place. It would sometimes move around my chest, and later it would move towards my stomach. At the end of June, I could not get to sleep after I felt it. As I began to feel the discomfort at the end of the evening, I went for a glass of sweet honey and herbal tea to soothe my pain and attempted to complete some work on my computer until I felt no pain. It was often longer than two hours before I fell into sleep. Yet I continued with my hectic schedule. I was thinking that a 3 km run every early morning, some herbal tea, and a healthy foods would suffice to alleviate the pain I felt. Then, I realized that none of these things worked.

I would regularly send Good Energy Healing hugs, Love and Good Luck to my Facebook friends however I did not take the time to get myself healed.

Our family's pet, an angel called Gosha was diagnosed with a problem in his eye. The eye wouldn't even be able to open. I offered him a healing energy, and also asked my Facebook buddies to aid him. A majority of them offered prayer and energy for healing for Gosha's eye, which got healed quickly.

And I never asked my Facebook buddies to aid me. Also, I didn't spend the opportunity to heal myself.

Gosha's eye healed however my pains got more and more intense. I fell asleep much less in the evening as I began to weaken and weaken.

The summer months are here. It was time to leave for Europe. My back was hurting throughout the restless night prior to when we set off for our travels and on the day following, while making final planning. The pain continued to linger on my lengthy and sleepless plane ride to Europe and was there for me through that packed first day.

I could have gone for over 24 hours without sleeping. This was an extremely difficult period. The following three weeks were filled with interesting activities and events, however there was no way to get sufficient sleep. My body was aching and the pains in my body would wake me up at night time repeatedly.

Each week, I sent LIGHT and Love as well as healing energy as well as Good Luck to a lot of my Facebook friends however, I did not take the time to give Love for me.

My energy was not as high as my typical energy and this affected our sales of art. This made me nervous and scared, making my health worse. After three weeks off I came home exhausted and the pains got more severe.

2. The first attempt to heal me.

After returning from my trip, my health was in a very bad state. Night pains was becoming chronic, and I was six kilograms less than my usual weight. I came to the realization that I had to take care of my own health. I set out on a new plan with positive affirmations, exercising and eating healthy.

I'd be sure to repeat these affirmations to the world at dawn:

I'm secure

I'm content.

I'm well

I'm comfortable.

It's as simple as that.

It was my first time walking two to three km each morning before eating breakfast.

I prepared a unique herbal tea made of Saint-John's-wort, mint, chamomile as well as valerian root, ground fennel seeds Echinacea as well as honey. I took a sip when I was feeling a bit hurt and around 1.5 Liters throughout every meal. I ensured that I was eating only food that was healthy.

Additionally, I started using an instrument I designed myself to aid in the purpose of balancing energy. It transmits electric impulses at acupuncture points.

These steps for healing have been helpful to me previously. However, this time, even after about a week of treatment it was not a significant improvement.

I was terrified. I contacted my family physician. The doctor's secretary inquired about my symptoms, and then made an appointment. On the next day, I received an urgent call from the office of a doctor advising me to go straight in the hospital.

I wasn't going there. It was then that I thought about how I endured a full day in the hospital, waiting in line to receive treatment for bleeding injuries from a bike accident. Instead, I chose to get the assistance of an expert energy healer.

4. The experimentation of different healing methods

The way forward

Between September 2014 and February 2015, I attempted a variety of methods to help me heal. There were times when things would go well for several days, or perhaps for a week. But at night, my pain would be back. until I came across a magical solution. Continue reading. We'll let you know soon.

4.1 Spiritual DNA, Innate method

The majority of scientists speak about DNA in a biochemical perspective viewpoint without taking into account biophysical aspects. According to esoteric doctrines DNA also has a the quantum, vibrational nature. Many call it Quantum DNA, Spiritual DNA, Soul DNA or Innate. Learn more details about Spiritual DNA on the website of Dr. John Ryan's work "The Missing Pill" [66.

In Lee Carol's channelings to Kryon [2,3I learned that we could reprogram our DNA to live a long healthy and happy life through communicating through the spiritual DNA.

Then I sat in meditation on my Spiritual DNA, and prayed to reprogram it in order to become healthful and balanced, allowing me to live a an extended life and an active process of growth. However however, I experienced pain in the evenings. Was it because I wasn't properly connected during the reconfiguring? I was thinking. Then in the book, you'll find out the best way to determine the relationship to Your Spiritual DNA.

On January 7, 2015, I realized it may be something I been handed down by my father, who also had issues. Then I sat in meditation, connected to Spiritual DNA, and asked them for a reprogramming of my DNA to rid me of inheritable issues.

On the 9th January in my 5km exercise, I was looking back at the past and future and not enjoying the lovely warm day at the moment.

My awareness was switched. The fresh air was revitalizing me. I felt joy. It radiated through my body and around me after which to the present. I received an inner strong affirmation that I did not need to travel anywhere in order to be joyous. The joy I feel is always within me, waiting to be brought out and be invited into my now.

The 11th of January, I had this conversation about my spiritual DNA. It's not easy to believe, but you have to open up. I applied the process of kinesiology to talk with my Spiritual DNA. Learn the method.

4.2 Applied Kinesiology (AK) or techniques for testing muscles

George J. Goodheart, chiropractor, developed an applied kinesiology practice in the year 1964, and then began to teach this technique to other chiropractors [44. Although this technique is mostly employed by chiropractors, it's being used by other doctors currently, like the treatment of allergies. Some people are skeptical of how effective it is until they've done it for themselves and observed the outcomes. Applied Kinesiology, also known as an exercise testing method, is a technique to extract data from your unconscious.

There are many methods to choose from. A few methods you could employ to evaluate yourself are:

* Hand Solo Method

* Falling Log Method

* Hole-In-One Method

* Linked Rings Method

* Thumping on Thymus Method

* Pendulum

* Sway Test

Learn more about the various techniques in the Heal Yourself book [14].

I tested a number of these strategies over a span that was 6 months. I did not get the same results from all of these methods. However, I did find one that is very effective for me: the Sway Test. I discovered it through Dianne Nassr, when I was the host of at the "Healing with Lightworkers" telesummit 11The 11th. This telesummit had incredible healing tips, however this technique has changed my life. Since then I've only used this technique since I've found that it provides me with the best results.

4.3 Utilizing the Sway Test

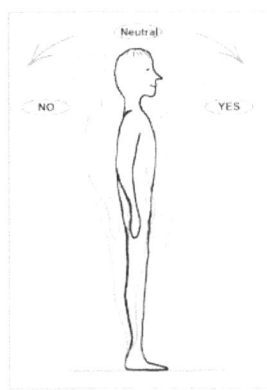

The sway test can be considered one of the easiest and most efficient ways to gain answers to your unconscious mind spiritual DNA, as well as your Higher Self. It does not require the aid from any other person. It is necessary to stand in order in order to utilize it (see fig.1) Also, it requires a little more time to complete than others self-testing techniques.

Fig. 1. Sway test.

Preparation

Utilize the steps listed below to help you prepare for the sway exam:

1. Take a break in a space that is free of distractions like the television and music.

I find it to work most effectively when I'm at home however, you can perform the exercise with someone else who would be willing to share the experience with you.

2. Keep your posture steady, keeping your feet spread shoulder-width separated for equilibrium and keep your hands to your edges.

Certain descriptions of this approach suggest facing North However, according to my own experience I've found that this method works regardless of direction.

3. Take a break from all your worries and let your body relax. If you are comfortable doing so, close your eyes. If you have trouble to keep the eyes shut, then doing the same thing with your eyes open is fine too.

4. Imagine that the golden white light beam links 3 locations within your body: The heart area, chakra of the heart as well as your crown chakra. Check out fig.2.

My own variation to the traditional approach. If you're only beginning to learn about the sway method You could leave out this part, however, I have found that when I apply it, I achieve better results.

5. Make a hand gesture as you visualize the light beam (step 4.). (This is one of my modifications to the traditional method however, it's not required.) You can slowly bind your fingers in a tight knot, with the tips reaching out and upwards. Check out fig.3. The technique can be done by using your left or the right hand or use both hands simultaneously. Personally, I like doing this using both hands at once.

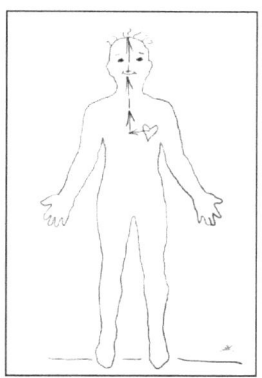

Fig.2. Imagine a golden white light beam connecting 3 points, my heart, my heart chakra as well as the chakra of crown.

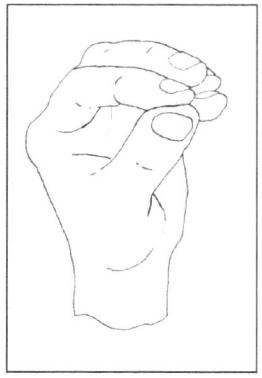

Fig.3. Balance gesture.

The hand gesture represents connection to Spiritual DNA as well as the balance. It was my experience that after a few hours of practice I was able to perform the motion to make links with my spiritual DNA almost instantaneously. If you're just beginning to master the sway method You could leave it out.

You can also employ a different mudra or gesture such as or the Gyan Mudra, known as the mudra of wisdom. Check out fig.4. Make sure to touch the thumb with the tip of your index finger using the remaining three fingers extended. This helps to increase memory and improves brain function. It improves focus and reduces the risk of insomnia. Many people use the gesture to make a good impression. You'll notice that your body continuously changes its posture and in various directions, as your muscles try to maintain your in balance. The movements are quite subtle and not noticeable because they're not under your conscious command.

3. Energy healers can help you.

The middle of August, I made the decision to seek out a good energy healer. I am a huge fan of the book "Energy Medicine", by Donna Eden [1]. I wanted to find someone in the area who practices Donna's techniques for energy healing. Through the Internet I discovered one in my area. She was trained by Donna who was also accredited by Donna to do energy healing. The next day, I was able to have a great 90 minute energy therapy session which greatly helped me. Following that exercise, I got an enjoyable night's sleep in the very first night in a long time. I was so content. The joy was short-lived. Within a few weeks it was back to the same pain.

I realized that only by applying my own power can be able to heal myself. Also, I must get rid of what caused the problem to prevent it from recurring.

Chapter 13: Conduct the testing of sway

Conduct the sway test by following these instructions:

1. Be aware of your efforts to talk with your spiritual DNA. In your mind, say "I'm connected to my Spiritual DNA."

2. For a test to determine if you've got the connection, speak out an item that you are certain is true to 100 such as, "My name is ". In my instance I'll tell you "My name is Alexander".

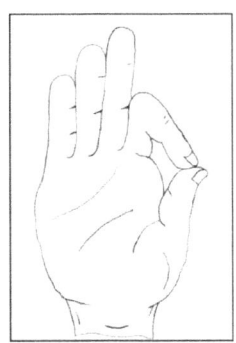

Fig.4. Gyan Mudra the mudra of information.

Your subconscious mind, or Spiritual DNA, a chance to communicate to you this way. The subconscious mind of your Spiritual DNA, knows what's truthful. When you affirm a affirmation, your body is able to move towards the future, as the body's inclination is towards honesty and positivity. Your body is likely to move forward in a noticeable manner in a matter of minutes. This means that you are YES.

3. Always test the connection to the connection with Spiritual DNA. Use an untrue assertion For example "my name is ". In my instance, I'll tell you "My name is Elena". In the event that you pick an identity that's not yours Your subconscious mind will recognize that the statement doesn't hold any truth. The body's posture will change within just a few minutes. This means that you are NOT.

4. "Neutral" or "Neutral" to have your body return to a neutral posture. It is done in between inquiries. My own variation to the conventional technique. I have found that it makes outcomes more stable.

5. You can repeat the true and false tests that you have learned in the earlier procedures several times, randomly so that you can be sure you're getting accurate outcomes prior to asking the inquiry to which you're seeking the answer.

6. Declare "I'm connected to my Spiritual DNA". Your body is likely to move forward in a noticeable manner in a matter of minutes. This indicates that you're prepared to interact to your spiritual DNA.

7. You are now ready to answer your inquiry. Make sure to ask your inquiry in a way which can be responded to using only "Yes" or "No." When your body is leaning

forward, it will answer "Yes," but if you lean backwards, then it is "No."

A few tips to get answers that are more trustworthy:

Let your body move in its own way. Do not try to force it. Be patient! Do it every day by asking questions for which you have the answer already. If you can answer them with confidence, and you're ready to tackle other questions. The body's reaction time will decrease dramatically after your daily practice of many weeks.

* If you're asking questions, ensure that your brain is uncluttered by other thoughts. Keep your attention on the issue that you're attempting to ask. If you are letting your mind wander or tangling, it may be hard to the subconscious brain, or your spiritual DNA to pinpoint exactly what you're actually asking. If, for instance when you ask a question, your mind

immediately starts thinking about the disagreement you had recently with a person? The chances are that you'll start to revert back, as your memory of the incident is negative and the body naturally wants to disengage from the event.

* If you're going to answer a lot of questions, or your test takes longer than usual It's best to check your baseline regularly. Choose a test for which you have the right solution, like the name of your friend and another name. If you receive the correct answer, you can continue the session.

• Allow love to overflow your heart. Don't think of your self negatively.

Make sure you have your questions prepared carefully. The language of the question must be precise. It is essential that the questions are responded to using "Yes" or "No".

It is important to ensure that you're hydrated! Sipping a glass of water 15 to 20 minutes before your session can prove very beneficial.

If you're unable to utilize the sway technique, then try alternatives listed on the 7th page. Explore them until you have which one is the best suited and most reliable for your needs.

My wife Elena employs her personal method. It's called the Shifting Method of the Energy Ball. Elena said that whenever she's feeling exhausted or bored, or requires a quick consult She thinks about talking to her spiritual DNA. She often does this while sleeping in a chair, or sitting down. No matter how she positions her body, it doesn't make a difference as long as you have a space where there are no distractions. An intense focus, a strong desire and the belief that all information comes from an uplifting and compassionate Source is essential. A relaxed, open and tolerant attitude is equally important.

Elena states that she can sense an energy ball dense in the solar plexus (about 5" large) in a response to a YES to the Spiritual DNA. When she says no, she feels an energy cloud within her back on the same level as her solar the plexus. The neutral point lies somewhere in the middle.

At times, she will focus her mind the identical tests for connecting that I use verbally. The test is similar to the following: